contents

Weight Watchers *Dining Out Companion* New for FlexPoints!

Welcome to Weight Watchers ***Dining Out Companion.*** This exciting edition, new for FlexPoints, is better than ever! With 33% more restaurants than ever before, and new ***POINTS***® values based on all the latest menu formulations, this guide is indispensible no matter what you crave. Whether it's a special event or a quick bite, with Weight Watchers ***Dining Out Companion,*** eating out can be a wonderful part of your weight-loss journey!

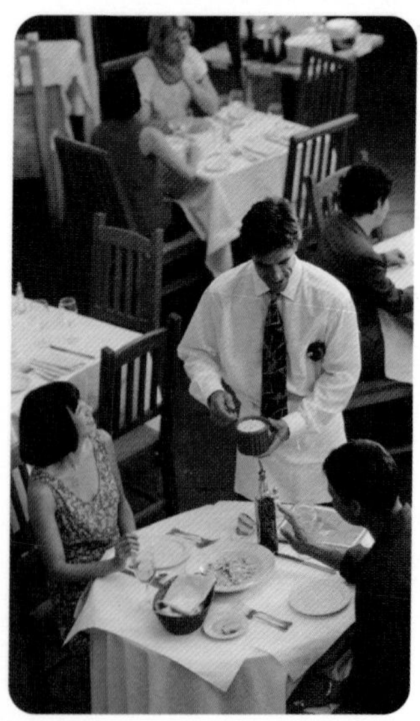

But this guide is more than just a Food List from popular restaurants. You'll also find…

- satisfying, new meal ideas that make planning easy,
- low-***POINT*** menu suggestions to help keep you at your ***POINTS*** Target,
- non-specific listings of foods from local restaurants, including ethnic favorites, and
- tips to help make eating out a successful part of your weight-loss experience.

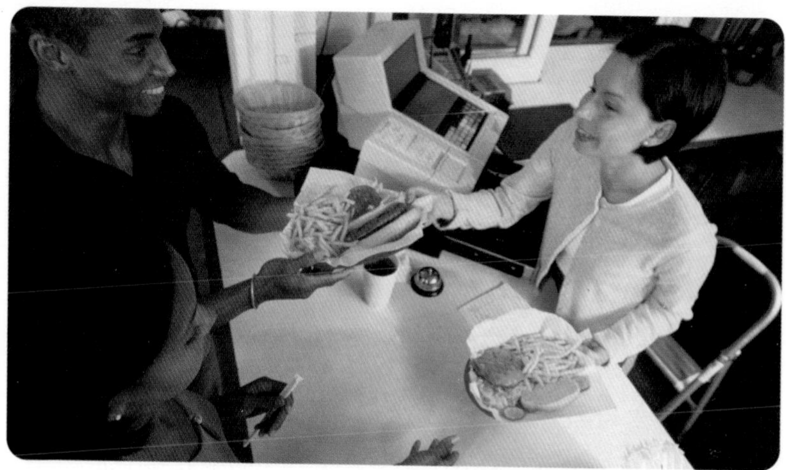

You can use Weight Watchers ***Dining Out Companion*** with confidence because the ***POINTS*** values for all foods listed were calculated by Weight Watchers International, Inc. from the most current nutrition information provided by the participating restaurants at the time of publication. However, since nutritional variations may occur based on portion control, ingredient selection, and other factors, for specific nutrition information as researched directly by the restaurants or independent third parties, please contact participating restaurants.

Keep in mind that a restaurant chain's offerings may vary by location. All items featured in each restaurant's menu listings and photograph may not be available at all locations.

As the world's leading name in weight loss, Weight Watchers is always here to help you reach your weight-loss goals. So enjoy eating out! Try somewhere new or visit an old favorite. With Weight Watchers *Dining Out Companion* the choice is up to you! Bon appétit!

diningout**tips**

- Make low-***POINT*** selections for your other meals during the day; you'll save ***POINTS*** to spend on eating out occasions.
- Plan in advance. Save some of your FlexPoints to use when eating out.
- Eat something light, such as a piece of fruit, a favorite vegetable, a small container of yogurt, or a mug of broth-based soup before going out to a meal.
- Take a few moments to decide what you want to order. Don't order hastily.
- Voice your needs to the waiter or order taker. They are generally able to accommodate menu changes when requested to do so.
- Look for lower-fat choices by focusing on words such as grilled, broiled, steamed, poached, or roasted.
- Drink water, unsweetened iced or hot tea or coffee, or a diet beverage during your meal to slow down your eating.
- Start your meal with a salad (with the dressing on the side!).
- Eat slowly and taste every mouthful. Put your fork down between bites. Take a break from eating to enjoy conversation with your dining companions.
- Listen closely to your body's signals. The goal is to eat only until you are no longer hungry.
- Use your ***Dining Out Companion*** to order meals that will help you keep at your ***POINTS*** Target. If an item has more ***POINTS*** than you'd like, share it with someone or pack up half a portion to take home and enjoy at another time.

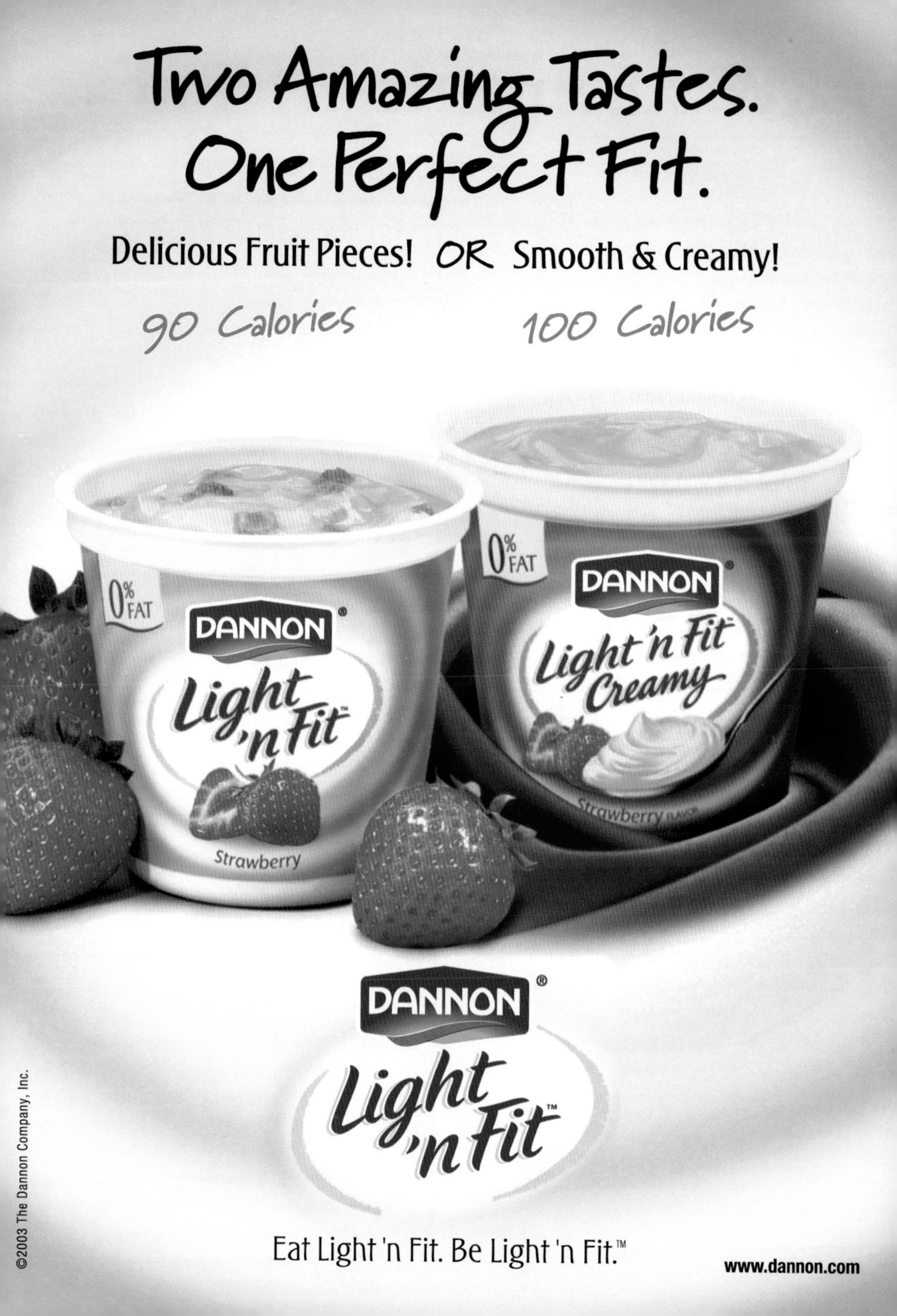
Two Amazing Tastes.
One Perfect Fit.
Delicious Fruit Pieces! OR Smooth & Creamy!
90 Calories
100 Calories
0% FAT
DANNON®
Light 'n Fit™
Strawberry
0% FAT
DANNON®
Light 'n Fit™
Creamy
Strawberry FLAVOR
DANNON®
Light 'n Fit™
Eat Light 'n Fit. Be Light 'n Fit.™
www.dannon.com
©2003 The Dannon Company, Inc.

A&W® All American Food™

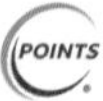

Burgers&Sandwiches

Jr. Hamburger, 1 10
Hamburger, 1 10
Deluxe Hamburger, 1 11
Jr. Cheeseburger, 1 11
Cheeseburger, 1 11
Deluxe Cheeseburger, 1 12
Deluxe Double Cheeseburger, 1 19
Deluxe Bacon Cheeseburger, 1 13
Deluxe Bacon Double Cheeseburger, 1 21
Grilled Chicken Sandwich, 1 6
Crispy Chicken Sandwich, 1 13
Hot Dog (plain), 1 7
Cheese Dog, 1 8
Coney (Chili) Dog, 1 7
Coney (Chili)/Cheese Dog, 1 8

Sides

Fries, 1 small serving 6
Fries, 1 large serving 9
Cheese Fries, 1 serving 8
Chili Fries, 1 serving 8
Chili/Cheese Fries, 1 serving 9
Onion Rings, 1 serving 8

MealIdeas

1 Grilled Chicken Sandwich
1 small serving Fries

1 Coney (Chili) Dog
1 small serving Fries

1 Grilled Chicken Sandwich
1 serving Onion Rings

ARBY'S®

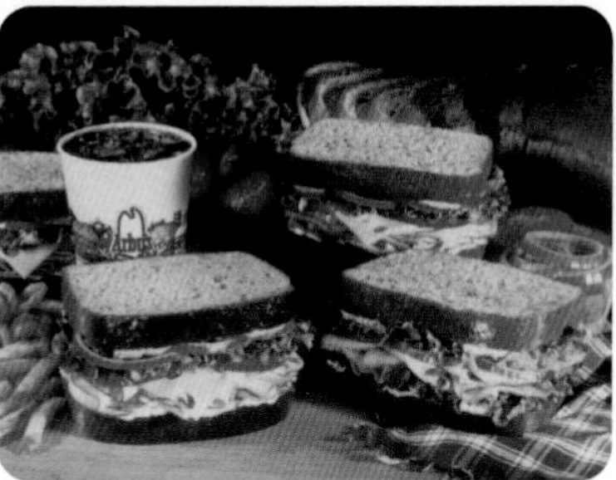

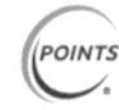

POINTS

Roast Beef Sandwiches

Item	POINTS
ARBY-Q® Sandwich, 1	8
ARBY'S® Melt with Cheddar Sandwich, 1	8
Beef 'N Cheddar Sandwich, 1	11
BIG MONTANA® Sandwich, 1	15
Giant Roast Beef Sandwich, 1	11
Junior Roast Beef Sandwich, 1	7
Regular Roast Beef Sandwich, 1	8
Super Roast Beef Sandwich, 1	11

Sub Sandwiches

Item	POINTS
French Dip Sub, 1	10
Hot Ham 'N Swiss Sub, 1	12
Italian Sub, 1	19
Philly Beef 'N Swiss Sub, 1	17
Roast Beef Sub, 1	19
Turkey Sub, 1	15

Light Sandwiches

Item	POINTS
Light Grilled Chicken Sandwich, 1	5
Light Roast Chicken Deluxe Sandwich, 1	5
Light Roast Turkey Deluxe Sandwich, 1	5

MARKETFRESH® Sandwiches

Item	POINTS
Roast Beef & Swiss Sandwich, 1	19
Roast Chicken Caesar Sandwich, 1	19
Roast Ham & Swiss Sandwich, 1	17
Roast Turkey & Swiss Sandwich, 1	17

Other Sandwiches

Item	POINTS
Chicken Breast Fillet Sandwich, 1	13
Chicken Cordon Bleu Sandwich, 1	15
Chicken, Bacon & Swiss Sandwich, 1	15
Grilled Chicken Deluxe Sandwich, 1	10
Hot Ham 'N Swiss Sandwich, 1	8
Roast Chicken Club Sandwich, 1	12

MARKETFRESH® Salads

(*POINTS* values include 2 saltine crackers & 1 crouton packet)

Item	POINTS
Caesar Salad, without dressing, 1	2
Caesar Side Salad, 1	1
Chicken Finger Salad, without dressing, 1	14
Grilled Chicken Caesar, without dressing, 1	5
Turkey Club Salad, without dressing, 1	8

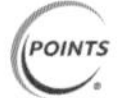

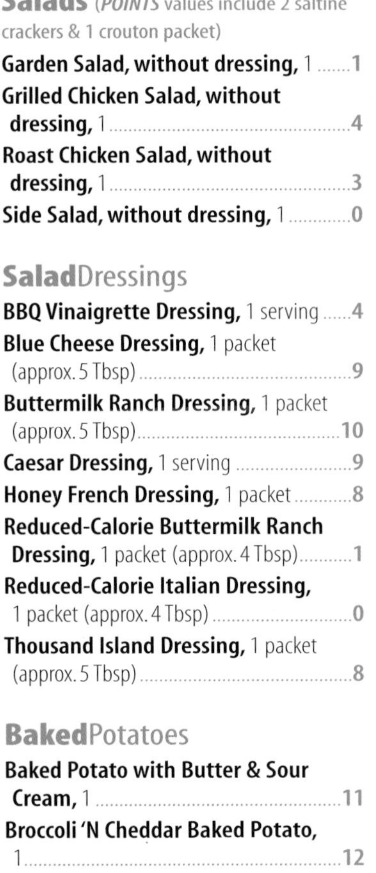

Salads (*POINTS* values include 2 saltine crackers & 1 crouton packet)

Garden Salad, without dressing, 1 1

Grilled Chicken Salad, without dressing, 1 4

Roast Chicken Salad, without dressing, 1 3

Side Salad, without dressing, 1 0

Salad Dressings

BBQ Vinaigrette Dressing, 1 serving 4

Blue Cheese Dressing, 1 packet (approx. 5 Tbsp) 9

Buttermilk Ranch Dressing, 1 packet (approx. 5 Tbsp) 10

Caesar Dressing, 1 serving 9

Honey French Dressing, 1 packet 8

Reduced-Calorie Buttermilk Ranch Dressing, 1 packet (approx. 4 Tbsp) 1

Reduced-Calorie Italian Dressing, 1 packet (approx. 4 Tbsp) 0

Thousand Island Dressing, 1 packet (approx. 5 Tbsp) 8

Baked Potatoes

Baked Potato with Butter & Sour Cream, 1 11

Broccoli 'N Cheddar Baked Potato, 1 12

Deluxe Baked Potato, 1 15

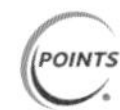

Chicken Fingers

Chicken Finger Snack, 1 serving 14

Chicken Finger, 4-pack, 1 serving 16

Dipping Sauces

BBQ Dipping Sauce, 1 packet 1

BRONCO BERRY SAUCE®, 1 packet 2

Honey Mustard Sauce, 1 serving 4

HORSEY SAUCE®, 1 packet 2

Marinara Sauce, 1 packet 1

TANGY SOUTHWEST SAUCE®, 1 packet 7

Fries & Sides

Curly Fries, 1 small serving 7

Curly Fries, 1 medium serving 9

Curly Fries, 1 large serving 14

Cheddar Curly Fries, 1 medium serving 10

Homestyle Fries, child-size, 1 serving 5

Homestyle Fries, 1 small serving 6

Homestyle Fries, 1 medium serving 8

Homestyle Fries, 1 large serving 12

JALAPEÑO BITES®, 1 serving 8

Mozzarella Sticks, 1 serving 11

Onion Petals, 1 serving 10

Potato Cakes, 2 pieces 6

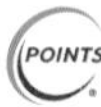

Breakfast

Biscuit with Butter, 2 7
Biscuit with Bacon, 1 8
Biscuit with Ham, 1 8
Biscuit with Sausage, 1 11
Croissant with Bacon, 1 8
Croissant with Ham, 1 8
Croissant with Sausage, 1 11
French-Toastix, without powdered sugar and syrup, 6 pieces 8
Maple Syrup, 1 serving (3 Tbsp) 3
Sourdough with Bacon, 1 8
Sourdough with Ham, 1 8
Sourdough with Sausage, 1 11
Swiss Cheese, 1 slice 1

Shakes

Chocolate Shake, 1 regular 11
Jamocha Shake, 1 regular 11
Vanilla Shake, 1 regular 11

Desserts

Apple Turnover, with icing, 1 9
Cherry Turnover, with icing, 1 9

Note: All items are not carried in all locations. Check with individual restaurants for any menu clarification.

MealIdeas

1 Grilled Chicken Salad with
1 packet Croutons and
1 packet Reduced-Calorie Italian Dressing
2 Saltine Crackers

1 Light Roast Turkey Deluxe Sandwich
1 Garden Salad with
1 packet Croutons and
1 packet Reduced-Calorie Italian Dressing
2 Saltines

1 Hot Ham 'N Swiss Sandwich
1 Caesar Side Salad with
1 packet Croutons and
1 packet Reduced-Calorie Italian Dressing
2 Saltine Crackers

Atlanta Bread Company®

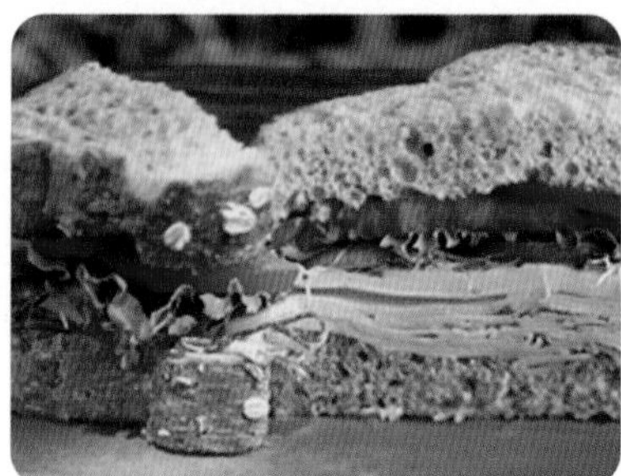

Soup

Black Bean & Ham, 1 cup 4
Chicken Chil, 1 cup 4
Chicken Gumbo Soup, 1 cup 2
Chicken Noodle, 1 cup 2
Chicken & Dumplings, 1 cup 6
Chicken Tortilla, 1 cup 3
Clam Chowder, 1 cup 7
Classic Beef Chili, 1 cup 6
Cream of Baked Potato Soup, 1 cup 5
Cream of Broccoli, 1 cup 4
French Onion, 1 cup 1
Garden Vegetable, 1 cup 1
Italian Wedding Soup, 1 cup 2
Lentil with Roasted Garlic Soup, 1 cup 3
Mushroom, Barley & Sage Soup, 1 cup 1
Pasta Fagioli, 1 cup 3
Seven Bean & Ham, 1 cup 5
Southwestern Chicken, 1 cup 4
Spicy Black Bean & Rice Soup, 1 cup 2
Szechuan Hot & Sour Soup, 1 cup 2
Tomato Florentine, 1 cup 2
Tomato with Fennel & Dill Soup, 1 cup 2
Vegetable Chili, 1 cup 3
Wisconsin Style Cheese, 1 cup 5

Sandwiches

ABC Special Sandwich, 1 9
Avocado Sandwich, 1 14
Bella Basil Chicken Sandwich, 1 18
Chargrilled Chicken Pesto Panini Sandwich, 1 17
Chicken Cordon Bleu Panini, 1 12
Chicken Salad Sandwich, 1 14
Cuban Pork Loin Panini, 1 17
Curry Chicken Salad Sandwich, 1 14
Honey Maple Ham Sandwich, 1 6
Italian Vegetarian Panini, 1 13
Pastrami Sandwich, 1 9
Roast Beef Sandwich, 1 9
Roasted Breast of Turkey Sandwich, 1 8
Tuna Salad Sandwich, 1 12
Turkey Club Panini, 1 18

Salads

Caesar Salad with Chicken, 1 7
Caesar Salad, 1 5
Chopstix Chicken Salad, without dressing, 1 11
Fruit Salad, 1 2
Greek Salad, with chicken, no dressing, no feta cheese, 1 5
House Salad, with chicken, 1 2
House Salad, without chicken, 1 0

POINTS®

SaladDressings

1000 Island Dressing, 2 Tbsp 4
Balsamic Vinaigrette, 1 serving 3
Caesar Dressing with Egg, 2 Tbsp 4
Fat Free Ranch, 2 Tbsp 0
Fat Free Raspberry Vinaigrette, 2 Tbsp 1
Greek Dressing, 2 Tbsp 3
Sesame Ginger Dressing, 1 oz 3

Breads&**Rolls**

Asiago Large, 1 serving 3
Asiago Strip, 1 serving 3
Cinnamon Raisin Loaf, 1 serving 3
Cracked Wheat, 1 serving 3
French Baguette, 1 serving 3
French Bread Strip, 1 serving 3
French Bread XL, 1 serving 3
French Rolls, 1 3
Honey Wheat, 1 serving 3
Nine Grain, 1 serving 3
Pumpernickel XL, 1 serving 3
Sourdough Baguette, 1 serving 3
Sourdough Loaf, 1 serving 3
Sourdough Rolls, 1 4
Sourdough Rye XL, 1 serving 3

POINTS®

Bagels

Asiago Bagel, 1 7
Blueberry Bagel, 1 7
Cinnamon Raisin Bagel, 1 6
Everything Bagel, 1 6
Honey Wheat Bagel, 1 6
Plain Bagel, 1 7
Poppy Seed Bagel, 1 6
Sesame Seed Bagel, 1 6

CreamCheese

Low Fat Chives Cream Cheese, 1 serving 1
Low Fat Honey Walnut Raisin Cream Cheese, 1 serving 2
Low Fat Veggie Cream Cheese, 1 serving 1

Croissants

Almond Croissant, 1 13
Apple Filled Croissant, 1 9
Cheese Croissant, 1 11
Chocolate Croissant, 1 14
French Croissant, 1 7
Raspberry/Cheese Croissant, 1 10

Danish

Apple Danish, 1 14
Cheese Danish, 1 15
Raspberry Cheese Danish, 1 15
Red Raspberry Danish, 1 14

Muffins

POINTS

- **Apple Cinnamon Muffin,** 1 9
- **Apple Muffin - Lowfat,** 1 6
- **Banana Muffin - Lowfat,** 1 6
- **Banana Walnut,** 1 10
- **Blueberry Muffin,** 1 10
- **Blueberry Muffin - Low Fat,** 1 6
- **Bran Raisin Muffin,** 1 10
- **Chocolate Chip Muffin,** 1 11
- **Chocolate Muffin - Low Fat,** 1 7
- **Cranberry Apple Muffin,** 1 9
- **Cranberry Orange Walnut Muffin,** 1 10
- **Lemon Poppy Seed,** 1 11
- **Mocha Chocolate Chip,** 1 11
- **Peaches & Creme Muffin,** 1 12
- **Pumpkin Muffin - Low Fat,** 1 6
- **Pumpkin Muffin,** 1 8
- **Zucchini Muffin,** 1 11

Muffin Tops

- **Banana Walnut Muffin Top,** 1 top 5
- **Blueberry Muffin Top,** 1 top 5
- **Chocolate Chip Muffin Top,** 1 top 5
- **Mocha Muffin Top,** 1 top 6
- **Pumpkin Muffin Top,** 1 top 4

Scones

- **Cranberry Scone,** 1 6
- **Lemon Scone,** 1 7
- **Maple Oat Walnut Scone,** 1 8
- **Raspberry Scone,** 1 8

POINTS

Cheesecake

- **Bailey's Cheesecake,** 1 slice 14
- **Cappuccino Cheesecake,** 1 slice 14
- **Pecan Turtle Cheesecake,** 1 slice 15
- **Snickers Cheesecake,** 1 slice 10

Cookies

- **Chocolate Chunk Cookie,** 1 9
- **Oatmeal Raisin Cookie,** 1 8
- **Peanut Butter Cookie,** 1 10
- **Shortbread Cookie,** 1 9
- **Triple Chocolate Chunk Cookie,** 1 5
- **White Chocolate Macadamia Nut,** 1 10

Miscellaneous Items

- **Croutons,** 1 serving 1
- **Dill Sauce,** 1 serving 1

Smoothies

- **Heath Coffee Cafechillo,** 1 5
- **Kona Mocha Coffee Cafechillo,** 1 5
- **Pineapple Mango Banana Smoothie,** 1 4
- **Spiced Chai Tea Cafechillo,** 1 3
- **Strawberry & Banana Smoothie,** 1 4
- **Strawberry Banana Blueberry Smoothie,** 1 4
- **Vanilla Latte Coffee Cafechillo,** 1 5

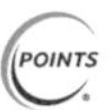

SpecialtySweets

Austrian Pretzel, 1 13
Bearclaw, 1 11
Chocolate Brownies (without walnuts), 1 11
Cinnamon Raisin Nut Roll, 1 18
Cinnamon Roll, 1 15
Eclair, 1 3
Sticky Bun, 1 11

Syrup

Almond Syrup, 1 serving 2
Caramel Syrup, 1 serving 2
French Vanilla Syrup, 1 serving 1
Hazelnut Syrup, 1 serving 2
Praline Syrup, 1 serving 2

CoffeeDrinks

House Latte, 1 short (12 fl oz) 5
House Latte, 1 tall (16 fl oz) 8
House Latte, 1 grande (20 fl oz) 10

MealIdeas

1 cup French Onion Soup with 1 serving Croutons
1 House Salad (with chicken) with Fat Free Ranch Dressing

1 cup Mushroom, Barley & Sage Soup
1 Caesar Salad with 1 serving Croutons

1 cup Garden Vegetable Soup
1 Poppy Seed Bagel with 1 serving Low Fat Veggie Cream Cheese

Au Bon Pain®

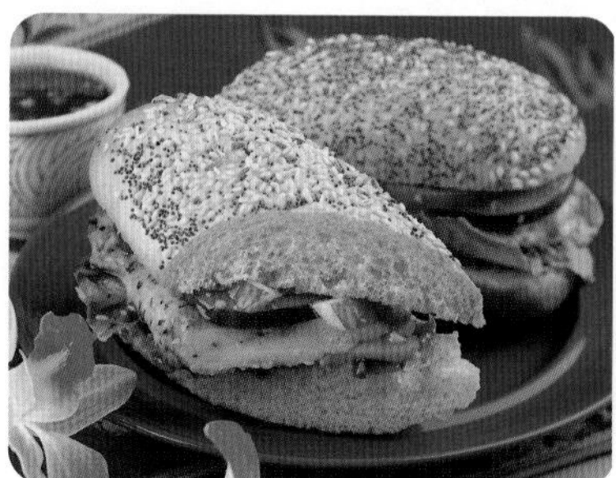

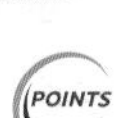

Soups

Black Bean, 1 medium (12 oz) ... 5
Black Bean, 1 large (16 oz) ... 6
Broccoli Cheddar, 1 medium (12 oz) ... 9
Broccoli Cheddar, 1 large (16 oz) ... 12
Chicken Florentine, 1 medium (12 oz) ... 6
Chicken Florentine, 1 large (16 oz) ... 8
Chicken Noodle Soup, 1 medium (12 oz) ... 3
Chicken Noodle Soup, 1 large (16 oz) ... 4
Clam Chowder, 1 medium (12 oz) ... 8
Clam Chowder, 1 large (16 oz) ... 11
Corn and Green Chili Bisque, 1 medium (12 oz) ... 5
Corn and Green Chili Bisque, 1 large (16 oz) ... 7
Corn Chowder, 1 medium (12 oz) ... 8
Corn Chowder, 1 large (16 oz) ... 11
Curried Rice & Lentil, 1 medium (12 oz) ... 2
Curried Rice & Lentil, 1 large (16 oz) ... 3
French Moroccan Tomato Lentil, 1 medium (12 oz) ... 3
French Moroccan Tomato Lentil, 1 large (16 oz) ... 4
Garden Vegetable Soup, 1 medium (12 oz) ... 1
Garden Vegetable Soup, 1 large (16 oz) ... 1
Lobster Bisque, 1 medium (12 oz) ... 9
Lobster Bisque, 1 large (16 oz) ... 10
Old Fashioned Tomato, 1 medium (12 oz) ... 4
Old Fashioned Tomato, 1 large (16 oz) ... 5
Pasta e fagioli, 1 medium (12 oz) ... 4
Pasta e fagioli, 1 large (16 oz) ... 6
Potato Cheese Soup, 1 medium (12 oz) ... 6
Potato Cheese Soup, 1 large (16 oz) ... 8
Potato Leek, 1 medium (12 oz) ... 7
Potato Leek, 1 large (16 oz) ... 7
Red Beans, Rice & Sausage, 1 medium (12 oz) ... 5
Red Beans, Rice & Sausage, 1 large (16 oz) ... 7
Reduced Sodium Mediterranean, 1 medium (12 oz) ... 5
Reduced Sodium Mediterranean, 1 large (16 oz) ... 7
Reduced Sodium Southwest Vegetable, 1 medium (12 oz) ... 4
Reduced Sodium Southwest Vegetable, 1 large (16 oz) ... 5
Southern Black Eyed Pea, 1 medium (12 oz) ... 5
Southern Black Eyed Pea, 1 large (16 oz) ... 7
Southwest Chicken Tortilla Soup, 1 medium (12 oz) ... 4

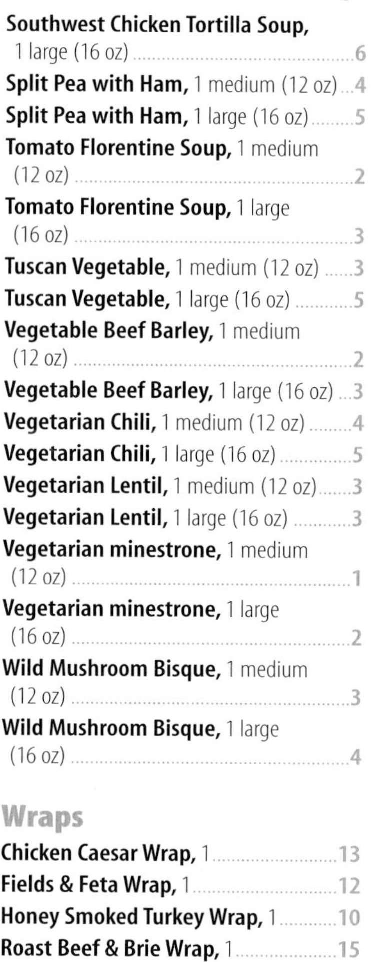

POINTS

Southwest Chicken Tortilla Soup, 1 large (16 oz) ... 6
Split Pea with Ham, 1 medium (12 oz) ... 4
Split Pea with Ham, 1 large (16 oz) ... 5
Tomato Florentine Soup, 1 medium (12 oz) ... 2
Tomato Florentine Soup, 1 large (16 oz) ... 3
Tuscan Vegetable, 1 medium (12 oz) ... 3
Tuscan Vegetable, 1 large (16 oz) ... 5
Vegetable Beef Barley, 1 medium (12 oz) ... 2
Vegetable Beef Barley, 1 large (16 oz) ... 3
Vegetarian Chili, 1 medium (12 oz) ... 4
Vegetarian Chili, 1 large (16 oz) ... 5
Vegetarian Lentil, 1 medium (12 oz) ... 3
Vegetarian Lentil, 1 large (16 oz) ... 3
Vegetarian minestrone, 1 medium (12 oz) ... 1
Vegetarian minestrone, 1 large (16 oz) ... 2
Wild Mushroom Bisque, 1 medium (12 oz) ... 3
Wild Mushroom Bisque, 1 large (16 oz) ... 4

Wraps

Chicken Caesar Wrap, 1 ... 13
Fields & Feta Wrap, 1 ... 12
Honey Smoked Turkey Wrap, 1 ... 10
Roast Beef & Brie Wrap, 1 ... 15
Southwestern Tuna Wrap, 1 ... 16

POINTS

Sandwiches

Arizona Chicken Sandwich, 1 ... 12
Cheese Sandwich, 1 ... 14
Chicken & Mozzarella Focaccia, 1 ... 19
Chicken Fo-Ca-Cha-Cha Sandwich, 1 ... 15
Chicken Tarragon with Field Greens, 1 ... 19
Fresh Mozzarella, Tomato & Pesto Sandwich, 1 ... 19
Garden Vegetable, Goat Cheese with Artichoke Topenade, 1 ... 12
Ham Sandwich, 1 ... 9
Hickory Smoked Ham & Brie, 1 ... 14
Honey Dijon Chicken Sandwich, 1 ... 16
Hot Grilled Chicken, 1 ... 14
Hot Roast Turkey Sandwich, 1 ... 11
Hot Roast Turkey, 1 ... 11
Hot Roasted Turkey Club Sandwich, 1 ... 14
Pane Bagniate, 1 ... 15
Roast Beef Sandwich, 1 ... 12
Smoked Turkey & Swiss with Cilantro Aioli, 1 ... 19
Smoked Turkey Sandwich, 1 ... 11
Thai Chicken Sandwich, 1 ... 10
Tuna Sandwich, 1 ... 12

POINTS

Fresh Rolls, Bread Stick & Bread Bowl

Baguette, 1 13
Braided Sandwich Roll with Topping, 1 9
Bread Stick, 1 4
Country White Sandwich Loaf, 1 2
Focaccia, 1 9
Four Grain Bread, 1 8
French Sandwich Roll, 1 5
Hearth Roll, 1 4
Multigrain Loaf, 1 2
Parisienne, 1 24
Petit Pain, 1 3
Soup Bread Bowl, 1 11
Tomato Herb Sandwich Loaf, 1 2

Fresh Salads (without dressing)

Caesar Salad, 1 5
Charbroiled Salmon Filet, 1 9
Chef's Salad, 1 6
Chicken Caesar Salad, 1 8
Chicken Oriental Salad, 1 4
Chicken Pesto Salad, 1 10
Cobb Salad, 1 17
Garden Salad, 1 3
Gorgonzola & Walnut Salad, 1 8
Mediterranean Chicken Salad, 1 7
Mozzarella & Red Pepper Salad, 1 9
Pear, Gorgonzola, Field Greens Salad, 1 8
Small Garden Salad, 1 1
Thai Chicken Salad, 1 8
Tomato, Mozzarella with Basil Pesto, 1 7
Tuna Salad, 1 serving 10

POINTS

Salad Dressings

Balsamic Vinaigrette, 1 serving 5
Bleu Cheese Dressing, 1 container 8
Buttermilk Ranch Dressing, 1 container 8
Caesar Dressing, 1 container 11
Fat Free Raspberry Dressing, 1 container 2
Lite Honey Mustard Dressing, 1 container 6
Lite Olive Oil Vinaigrette Dressing, 1 container 4
Lite Ranch Dressing, 1 container 7
Mandarin Orange Dressing, 1 serving 9
Mediterranean Dressing, 1 serving 2
Parmesan & Pepper Dressing, 1 container 11
Tarragon Mayonnaise Sauce, 1 serving 6
Thai Peanut Dressing, 1 container 3

Bagels (without spread)

Asiago Cheese Bagel, 1 7
Cinnamon Crisp Bagel with Topping, 1 11
Cinnamon Crisp Bagel, 1 7
Cinnamon Raisin Bagel, 1 5
Dutch Apple Bagel, 1 7
Everything Bagel, 1 6
Focaccia Bagel, 1 6
Honey 9 Grain Bagel, 1 6
Jalapeño Double Cheddar Bagel, 1 7
Onion Bagel, 1 6
Plain Bagel, 1 5
Poppy Seed Bagel, 1 6
Sesame Seed Bagel, 1 7

POINTS

Bagel Spreads

Plain Cream Cheese, 1 serving (4 Tbsp), 2 oz 5

Reduced Fat Cream Cheese, 1 serving (4 Tbsp), 2 oz 4

Reduced Fat Honey Walnut Cream Cheese, 1 serving (4 Tbsp), 2 oz 4

Reduced Fat Sun-Dried Tomato Cream Cheese, 1 serving (4 Tbsp), 2 oz 4

Reduced Fat Veggie Cream Cheese, 1 serving (4 Tbsp), 2 oz 4

Sundried Tomato Spread, 1 serving 2

Bagel Sandwiches

Egg on a Bagel Sandwich, 1 10

Egg on a Bagel with Bacon Sandwich, 1 12

Egg on a Bagel with Cheese & Bacon Sandwich, 1 14

Egg on a Bagel with Cheese Sandwich, 1 12

Fresh Fruit Cup

Fruit Cup, 1 small (8 oz) 1

Fruit Cup, 1 large (10 oz) 2

Plain and Flavored Yogurt

Blueberry Yogurt with Fresh Berries, 1 serving 4

Blueberry Yogurt with Granola, 1 serving 5

Plain Yogurt with Fresh Berries, 1 serving 4

POINTS

Plain Yogurt with Granola, 1 serving 5

Strawberry Yogurt with Fresh Berries, 1 serving 4

Strawberry Yogurt with Granola, 1 serving 5

Yogurt Parfait, 1 serving 12

Croissants

Almond Croissant, 1 11

Apple Croissant, 1 4

Chocolate Croissant, 1 7

Cinnamon Raisin Croissant, 1 6

Plain Croissant, 1 5

Raspberry Cheese Croissant, 1 6

Sweet Cheese Croissant, 1 7

Hot Croissants

Ham & Cheese Croissant, 1 6

Spinach & Cheese Croissant, 1 5

Gourmet Muffins

Banana Walnut Muffin, 1 10

Blueberry Muffin, 1 10

Bran Raisin Muffin, 1 8

Carrot Muffin, 1 12

Corn Muffin, 1 9

Cranberry Walnut Muffin, 1 12

Milk Chocolate Chunk Muffin, 1 12

Pumpkin Muffin, 1 11

Low Fat Muffins

Chocolate Cake Muffin, 1 5

Triple Berry Muffin, 1 5

POINTS

Cookies

½ Chocolate Shortbread Heart Cookie, 1 6
Chocolate Chip Cookie, 1 5
Chocolate Chunk Macadamia Nut Cookie, 1 6
English Toffee Cookie, 1 5
Gingerbread Man with Raisins & Icing, 1 6
Holiday Cookie with Icing & Sprinkles, 1 3
Oatmeal Raisin Cookie, 1 4
Peanut Butter Cookie, 1 5
Red Sugar Shortbread Heart Cookie, 1 6
Shortbread Cookie, 1 5
Walnut Raisin Cookie, 1 6

Dessert Bars

Blondie Brownie, 4 14
Cheese Cake Brownie, 4 11
Chocolate Chip Brownie, 4 11
Peanut Butter Brownie, 4 12
Pecan Brownie, 4 12

Danish & Baked Goods

Apple Cinnamon Pound Cake, 1 11
Apple Strudel, 1 piece 10
Banana Pear Pound Cake, 1 11
Cherry Strudel, 1 piece 9
Chocolate Crumb Cake, 1 18
Cinnamon Roll, 1 6
Cranberry Danish, 1 7
Creme de Fleur, 1 11

POINTS

Lemon Danish, 1 7
Pecan Roll, 1 14
Plain Crumb Cake, 1 19
Raspberry Crumb Cake, 1 18
Sweet Cheese Danish, 1 9

Scones

Chocolate Walnut Scone, 1 9
Cranberry Orange Almond Scone, 1 9
Maple Oat Pecan Date Scone, 1 9
Orange Scone, 1 8

Iced Specialty Drinks

Iced Cappuccino, 1 medium serving 4
Iced Cappuccino, 1 large serving 6
Peach Iced Tea, 1 medium serving 3
Peach Iced Tea, 1 large serving 3

Frozen Specialty Drink

Mocha Blast® Drink, 1 medium serving 8

MealIdeas

1 medium Chicken Noodle Soup
1 Spinach & Cheese Croissant

1 serving Blueberry Yogurt with Fresh Berries
1 Triple Berry Low Fat Muffin

1 small Fruit Cup
1 Cinnamon Raisin Bagel with 1 serving Reduced Fat Honey Walnut Cream Cheese

Auntie Anne's® Hand-Rolled Soft Pretzels

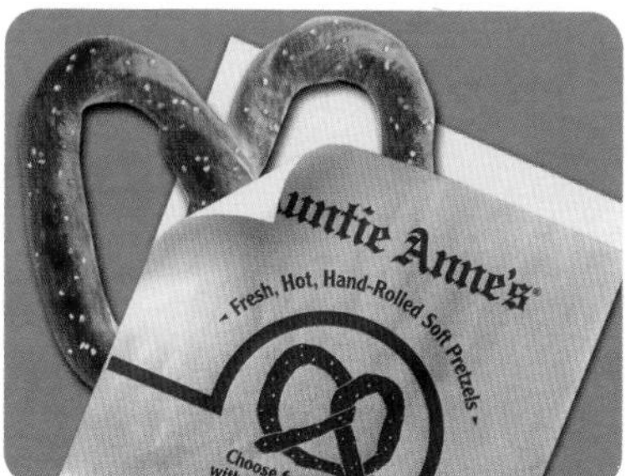

POINTS

Pretzels

Almond Pretzel, without butter, 1........7
Almond Pretzel, with butter, 1 8
Cinnamon Sugar Pretzel, without butter, 1 7
Cinnamon Sugar Pretzel, with butter, 1 9
Garlic Pretzel, without butter, 1............6
Garlic Pretzel, with butter, 1 7
Glazin' Raisin® Pretzel, without butter, 1 9
Glazin' Raisin® Pretzel, with butter, 1 10
Jalapeño Pretzel, without butter, 1 5
Jalapeño Pretzel, with butter, 1 6
Kidstix - Cinnamon Sugar, without butter, 4 5
Kidstix - Cinnamon Sugar, with butter, 4 6
KidStix - Original, without butter, 4.....4
KidStix - Original, with butter, 4 5
Original Pretzel, without butter, 1 6

POINTS

Original Pretzel, with butter, 1 7
Parmesan Herb Pretzel, without butter, 1 7
Parmesan Herb Pretzel, with butter, 1 9
Sesame Pretzel, without butter, 1 7
Sesame Pretzel, with butter, 1 8
Sour Cream & Onion, without butter, 1 6
Sour Cream & Onion, with butter, 1 7
Whole Wheat Pretzel, without butter, 1 6
Whole Wheat Pretzel, with butter, 1 7

DippingSauces

Caramel Dip, 1 serving 3
Cheese Sauce, 1 serving 3
Chocolate Flavored Dip, 1 serving 3
Hot Salsa Cheese, 1 serving 3
Light Cream Cheese, 1 serving 2
Marinara Sauce, 1 serving 0
Strawberry Cream Cheese, 1 serving 3
Sweet Mustard, 1 serving..........................1

DutchIce®

Blue Raspberry Dutch Ice®, 1 regular 3
Blue Raspberry Dutch Ice®, 1 large 5
Grape Dutch Ice®, 1 regular.......................4
Grape Dutch Ice®, 1 large 5
Kiwi-Banana Dutch Ice®, 1 regular..........4
Kiwi-Banana Dutch Ice®, 1 large 5

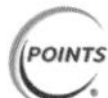

Lemonade Dutch Ice®, 1 regular..............6
Lemonade Dutch Ice®, 1 large..................9
Mocha Dutch Ice®, 1 regular.......................9
Mocha Dutch Ice®, 1 large.......................13
Orange Crème Dutch Ice®, 1 regular.......6
Orange Crème Dutch Ice®, 1 large..........8
Piña Colada Dutch Ice®, 1 regular............5
Piña Colada Dutch Ice®, 1 large...............7
Strawberry Dutch Ice®, 1 regular.............4
Strawberry Dutch Ice®, 1 large.................6
Wild Cherry Dutch Ice®, 1 regular............5
Wild Cherry Dutch Ice®, 1 large...............7

Some Low-*POINT* Ideas

each

4 Original Kidstix (without butter)
1 regular Grape, Kiwi-Banana, or Strawberry Dutch Ice®

each

1 Jalapeño Pretzel (without butter)
4 Cinnamon Sugar Kidstix (without butter)
4 Original Kidstix (with butter)
1 large Blue Raspberry, Grape, Kiwi-Banana, or Wild Cherry Dutch Ice®

each

1 Garlic, Original, Sour Cream & Onion, or Whole Wheat Pretzel (without butter)
1 Jalapeño Pretzel (with butter)
4 Cinnamon Sugar Kidstix (with butter)

Back Yard Burgers

POINTS

Classic Burgers

⅓ Lb. Back Yard Burger, 1 11
⅓ Lb. Back Yard Cheese Burger, 1 12
Great Little Burger®, 1 6

Signature ⅓ Lb. Specialty Burgers

Bacon Cheddar Burger, 1 16
Barbeque Bacon Burger, 1 16
Black Jack Burger, 1 14
Chili Cheese Burger, 1 14
Hawaiian Burger, 1 13
Miz Grazi's™ Burger, 1 13
Mushroom Swiss Burger, 1 13
Worcestershire Burger, 1 13

Chicken Sandwiches

Bacon Swiss Chicken Sandwich, 1 9
Barbeque Chicken Sandwich, 1 6
Blackened Chicken Sandwich, 1 6
Buffalo Ranch Chicken Sandwich, 1 13
Hawaiian Chicken Sandwich, 1 6
Honey Mustard Chicken Sandwich, 1 7
Lemon Butter Chicken Sandwich, 1 6
Savory Chicken Sandwich, 1 5

Back Yard Specialties

Back Yard BLT, 1 6
Back Yard Chili Cheese Dog, 1 10
Back Yard Chili Dog, 1 8
Back Yard Hot Dog, 1 8
Chicken Tenderloins, 3 pieces 10
Gardenburger®, 1 3

POINTS

Baked Potatoes & French Fries

Baked Potato, plain, 1 3
Chili and Cheddar Potato, 1 7
Miz Grazi's™ Chili Cheese Fries, 1 serving 8
Ranch Potato, 1 9
Salsa Potato, 1 5
Seasoned Fries, 1 regular 6
Waffle Fries, 1 regular 6

Dipping Sauces

Barbeque Dipping Sauce, 1 serving 1
Gourmet Dipping Sauce, 1 serving 4
Gravy Dipping Sauce, 1 serving 2
Honey Mustard Dipping Sauce, 1 serving 5

Salads

Blackened Chicken Salad, 1 3
Charbroiled Chicken Salad, 1 2
Garden Fresh Salad, 1 0

Salad Dressings

Fat Free Honey Dijon Dressing, 1 serving 1
Fat Free Italian Dressing, 1 serving 0
Fat Free Ranch Dressing, 1 serving 1
Honey Mustard Dressing, 1 serving 4
Italian Dressing, 1 serving 6
Ranch Dressing, 1 serving 8
Thousand Island Dressing, 1 serving 7

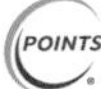

Cobblers

Apple Cobbler, 1 serving 10
Blackberry Cobbler, 1 serving 9
Cherry Cobbler, 1 serving 11
Peach Cobbler, 1 serving 10
Strawberry Cobbler, 1 serving 10

Ice Cream

Chocolate Milkshake, 1 13
Strawberry Milkshake, 1 13
Vanilla (scoop), 1 3
Vanilla Milkshake, 1 13

Meal Ideas

1 Gardenburger®
1 Garden Fresh Salad with
1 serving Fat Free Italian Dressing
1 scoop Vanilla Ice Cream

1 Savory Chicken Sandwich
1 Plain Baked Potato
1 Garden Fresh Salad with
1 serving Fat Free Italian Dressing

1 Great Little Burger®
1 Garden Fresh Salad with
1 serving Fat Free Ranch Dressing
1 scoop Vanilla Ice Cream

Baja Fresh Mexican Grill®

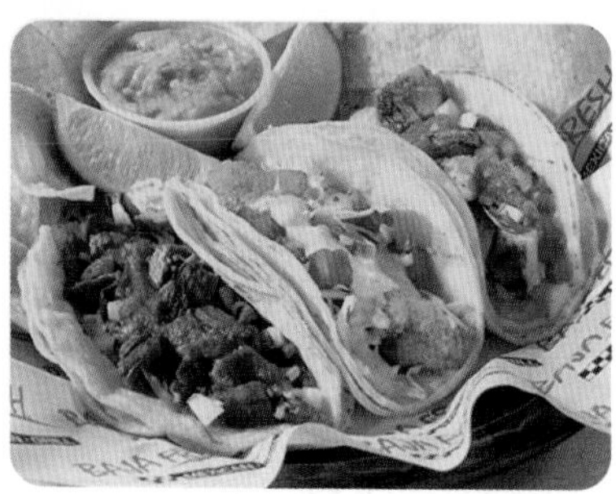

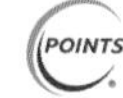

POINTS

Burritos

(without Chips and Sour Cream)

Baja Burrito with Charbroiled Chicken, 1 ... 18

Baja Burrito with Charbroiled Steak, 1 ... 21

Bean and Cheese Burrito (without Meat), 1 ... 19

Bean and Cheese Burrito with Charbroiled Chicken, 1 ... 22

Bean and Cheese Burrito with Charbroiled Steak, 1 ... 24

Burrito "Dos Manos" with Charbroiled Chicken, ½ ... 16

Burrito "Dos Manos" with Charbroiled Steak, ½ ... 17

Burrito Mexicano with Charbroiled Chicken, 1 ... 17

Burrito Mexicano with Charbroiled Steak, 1 ... 19

Burrito Ultimo with Charbroiled Chicken, 1 ... 19

Burrito Ultimo with Charbroiled Steak, 1 ... 21

POINTS

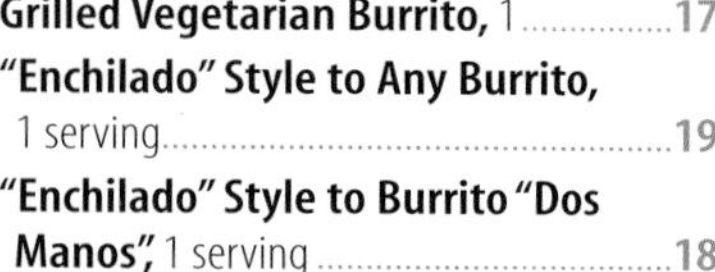

Grilled Vegetarian Burrito, 1 ... 17

"Enchilado" Style to Any Burrito, 1 serving ... 19

"Enchilado" Style to Burrito "Dos Manos", 1 serving ... 18

MexicanFavorites (without Chips)

Mini Quesa-dita™ with Charbroiled Chicken, 1 ... 18

Mini Quesa-dita™ with Charbroiled Steak, 1 ... 19

Mini Quesa-dita™ with Cheese, 1 ... 17

Mini Tosta-dita™ with Charbroiled Chicken, 1 ... 12

Mini Tosta-dita™ with Charbroiled Steak, 1 ... 14

Nachos with Charbroiled Chicken, 1 serving ... 48

Nachos with Charbroiled Steak, 1 serving ... 51

Nachos with Cheese, 1 serving ... 45

Quesadilla with Charbroiled Steak, 1 ... 36

Quesadilla with Charbroilled Chicken, 1 ... 34

Quesadilla with Cheese, 1 ... 31

Vegetarian Quesadilla, 1 ... 32

Specialties (without Chips)

Chicken Fajitas with Corn Tortillas, 1 serving ... 29

Chicken Fajitas with Flour Tortillas, 1 serving ... 33

Enchiladas Verdes with Charbroiled Chicken (without Sour Cream), 1 serving ... 19

POINTS

Enchiladas Verdes with Cheese (without Sour Cream), 1 serving 22
Vegetarian Enchiladas Verdes (without Sour Cream), 1 serving 18
Enchiladas with Charbroiled Chicken, 1 serving 20
Enchiladas with Charbroiled Steak, 1 serving 22
Enchiladas with Cheese, 1 serving 22
Steak Fajitas with Corn Tortillas, 1 serving 34
Steak Fajitas with Flour Tortillas, 1 serving 38

Tacos, Taquitos

"Baja Style" Taco - Charbroiled Chicken, 1 3
"Baja Style" Taco - Charbroiled Steak, 1 4
"Baja Style" Taco - Charbroiled Wild Gulf Shrimp, 1 4
"Baja" Fish Taco - Breaded Fish, 1 6
"Baja" Fish Taco - Charbroiled Fish, 1 ... 5
Charbroiled Chicken Taquitos with Beans, 1 serving 17
Charbroiled Chicken Taquitos with Rice, 1 serving 16
Charbroiled Steak Taquitos with beans, 1 serving 19
Charbroiled Steak Taquitos with Rice, 1 serving 19
Taco "Chilito" with Charbroiled Chicken, 1 serving 10
Taco "Chilito" with Charbroiled Steak, 1 serving 11

POINTS

Salads, Salad Dressings & Tostadas

Baja Ensalada with Charbroiled Chicken (without salad dressing), 1 ... 7
Baja Ensalada with Charbroiled Fish (without salad dressing), 1 8
Baja Ensalada with Charbroiled Steak (without salad dressing), 1 11
Side Salad (without salad dressing), 1 0
Tostada with Charbroiled Chicken, 1 26
Tostada with Charbroiled Steak, 1 29
Vegetarian Tostada, 1 24
Baja Dressing, 2 oz 9
Fat Free Salsa Verde Dressing, 2 oz 0
Ranch Dressing, 2 oz 6

Side Orders

Black Beans, 1 serving 7
Breaded Fish, 6 oz 9
Cebollitos, 12 pieces 0
Charbroiled Chicken, 6 oz 4
Charbroiled Fish, 6½ oz 4
Charbroiled Steak, 5 oz 8
Charbroiled Wild Gulf Shrimp, 5½ oz 3
Chips & "Salsa Baja"™, 1 serving 25
Gilled Onions, Peppers, & Chilies, 1 serving 1
Guacamole with Chips, 1 serving 32
Guacamole, 2 ounce side 1
Guacamole, 3 ounce side 2
Guacamole, 8 ounce side 4

Side Orders (con't) POINTS®

Pico de Gallo Salsa, 6 oz 0
Pinto Beans, 1 serving 6
Pronto Guacamole, 1 serving 13
Rice, 1 serving 5
Salsa Baja™, 2 ounce side 0
Salsa Baja™, 8 ounce side 1
Salsa Roja, 2 ounce side 0
Salsa Roja, 8 ounce side 1
Salsa Verde, 2 ounce side 0
Salsa Verde, 8 ounce side 0
Sour Cream, 1 side order 2

Tortillas

Corn Tortilla Chips, ½-oz serving 2
Corn Tortilla Chips, 1-oz serving 3
Corn Tortilla Strips, 1 serving 3
Corn Tortilla (with oil), 2 3
Corn Tortilla, 1 2
Flour Tortilla 8", 1 3
Mini Tostada Shell, 1 5
Tostada Shell, 1 11

MealIdeas

1 Charbroiled Chicken "Baja Style" Taco
1 Side Salad with
2 oz Fat Free Salsa Verde Dressing

1 Charbroiled Chicken "Baja Style" Taco
½-oz serving Corn Tortilla Chips with
2 oz side of Salsa Baja
1 Side Salad with
2 oz Fat Free Salsa Verde Dressing

5½ oz Charbroiled Wild Gulf Shrimp with 1 serving Rice
½-oz serving Corn Tortilla Chips with
2 oz side of Guacamole

Baskin-Robbins®

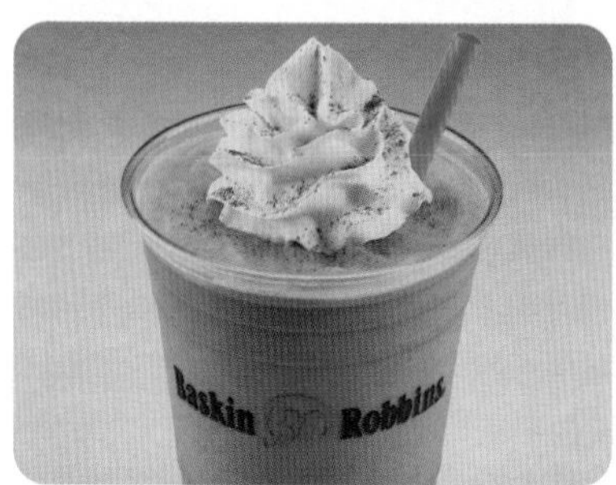

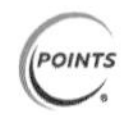

Deluxe Ice Cream

Chocolate Chip Cookie Dough, 2½ oz scoop (½ cup) 4

Chocolate Chip, 2½ oz scoop (½ cup) 4

Chocolate Fudge, 2½ oz scoop (½ cup) 4

Chocolate, 2½ oz scoop (½ cup) 4

French Vanilla, 2½ oz scoop (½ cup) 4

Gold Medal Ribbon, 2½ oz scoop (½ cup) 3

JAMOCA® Almond Fudge, 2½ oz scoop (½ cup) 4

JAMOCA®, 2½ oz scoop (½ cup) 3

Mint Chocolate Chip, 2½ oz scoop (½ cup) 4

Old Fashioned Butter Pecan, 2½ oz scoop (½ cup) 4

OREO® Cookies 'N Cream, 2½ oz scoop (½ cup) 4

Peanut Butter 'N Chocolate, 2½ oz scoop (½ cup) 4

Pistachio Almond, 2½ oz scoop (½ cup) 4

Pralines 'N Cream, 2½ oz scoop (½ cup) 4

POINTS

Rocky Road, 2½ oz scoop (½ cup) 4

Vanilla, 2½ oz scoop (½ cup) 3

Very Berry Strawberry, 2½ oz scoop (½ cup) 3

WORLD CLASS CHOCOLATE®, 2½ oz scoop (½ cup) 4

Sherbet

Blue Raspberry, 2½ oz scoop (½ cup) 3

Orange, 2½ oz scoop (½ cup) 3

Rainbow, 2½ oz scoop (½ cup) 3

Red Raspberry, 2½ oz scoop (½ cup) 3

Ices

Daiquiri, 2½ oz scoop (½ cup) 2

Lemon, 2½ oz scoop (½ cup) 2

Margarita, 2½ oz scoop (½ cup) 2

Watermelon, 2½ oz scoop (½ cup) 2

Low Fat Ice Cream

Divine Cherry Cheesecake, 1 2½ oz scoop (½ cup) 3

Espresso 'N Cream, 2½ oz scoop (½ cup) 2

No Sugar Added Ice Cream

Berries 'n Banana, 2½ oz scoop (½ cup) 1

Chocolate Chip, 2½ oz scoop (½ cup) 2

JAMOCA® Swiss Almond, 2½ oz scoop (½ cup) 2

Pineapple Coconut, 2½ oz scoop (½ cup) 2

Thin Mint Chip, 2½ oz scoop (½ cup) 2

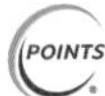

HardScoopYogurt (low-fat)

MAUI BROWNIE MADNESS®, 2½ oz scoop (½ cup) 3

RASPBERRY CHEESE LOUISE®, 2½ oz scoop (½ cup) 3

FountainDrinks

CAPPUCCINO BLAST™, with whipped topping, 1 7

CAPPUCCINO BLAST™, without whipped topping, 1 7

CHOCOLATE BLAST™, with whipped topping, 1 9

CHOCOLATE BLAST™, without whipped topping, 1 9

MOCHA CAPPUCCINO BLAST™, with whipped topping, 1 8

MOCHA CAPPUCCINO BLAST™, without whipped topping, 1 8

Nonfat CAPPUCCINO BLAST™, 1 4

Nonfat MOCHA CAPPUCCINO BLAST™, 1 5

Peach Smoothie, 1 7

Wild Berry Banana Smoothie, 1 8

Some Low-*POINT* Ideas

½ cup No Sugar Added Berries 'n Banana Ice Cream

each

½ cup Daiquiri, Lemon, Margarita, or Watermelon Ices

½ cup Low Fat Espresso 'N Cream Ice Cream

½ cup No Sugar Added Chocolate Chip, JAMOCA® Swiss Almond, Pineapple Coconut, or Thin Mint Chip Ice Cream

each

½ cup Deluxe Gold Medal Ribbon, JAMOCA®, or Very Berry Strawberry Ice Cream

½ cup Blue Raspberry, Orange, Rainbow, or Red Raspberry Sherbet

Big Boy®

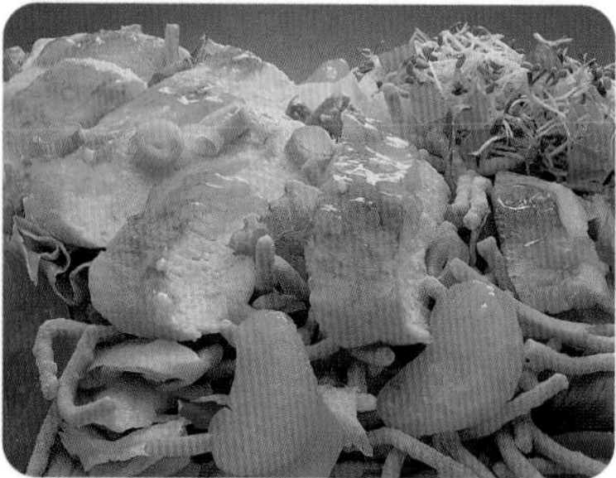

POINTS

Soup&Salads

Cabbage Soup, 1 bowl ... 1

Tossed Salad, without dressing, 1 ... 1

Grilled Chicken Breast Salad, with reduced-calorie ranch dressing, roll, and Promise® margarine, 1 ... 12

Oriental Chicken Breast Salad, with fat-free Oriental-sesame dressing, roll, and Promise® margarine, 1 ... 15

PitaPocketSandwiches

Chicken Breast with Mozzarella Pita, with reduced-calorie ranch dressing, 1 ... 11

Turkey pita, with reduced-calorie ranch dressing, 1 ... 8

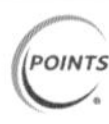

Dinners

Baked Cod, with tossed salad (no dressing), baked potato, roll, & Promise® margarine, 1 serving ... 17

Breast of Chicken with Mozzarella, with tossed salad (no dressing), baked potato, roll, and Promise® margarine, 1 serving ... 16

Cajun Cod, with tossed salad (no dressing), baked potato, roll, and Promise® margarine, 1 ... 17

Chicken 'n Vegetable Stir Fry, with tossed salad (no dressing), baked potato, roll, and Promise® margarine, 1 serving ... 17

Spaghetti Marinara, with tossed salad (no dressing), roll, and Promise® margarine, 1 serving ... 13

Vegetable Stir Fry, with tossed salad (no dressing), baked potato, roll, and Promise® margarine, 1 serving ... 13

Sides,DinnerRoll,& SaladDressings

Baked Potato, plain, 1 ... 3

Rice Pilaf, 1 serving ... 3

Dinner Roll, 1 ... 5

Promise® Margarine, 1 pat ... 1

Fat-Free Italian Dressing, 2 Tbsp ... 0

Fat-Free Oriental Dressing, 2 Tbsp ... 0

Reduced-Calorie Ranch Dressing, 2 Tbsp ... 1

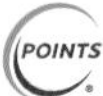

EggBeaters® Breakfast

Scrambled Egg Beaters®, with 2 slices of whole wheat toast and Promise® margarine, 1 serving 7

Plain Egg Beaters® Omelette, with 2 slices of whole wheat toast and Promise® margarine, 1 serving 7

Vegetarian Egg Beaters® Omelette, with 2 slices of whole wheat toast and Promise® margarine, 1 serving 7

Desserts

Fat Free Frozen Yogurt, 1 serving 2

Frozen Yogurt Shake, 1 3

Meal Ideas

1 bowl Cabbage Soup
1 Tossed Salad with
2 Tbsp Fat-Free Italian Dressing
1 serving Fat Free Frozen Yogurt

1 Vegetarian Egg Beaters® Omelette with 2 slices Whole Wheat Toast and Promise® Margarine

1 bowl Cabbage Soup
1 Turkey Pita Pocket Sandwich with Reduced-Calorie Ranch Dressing

BLIMPIE® Subs & Salads

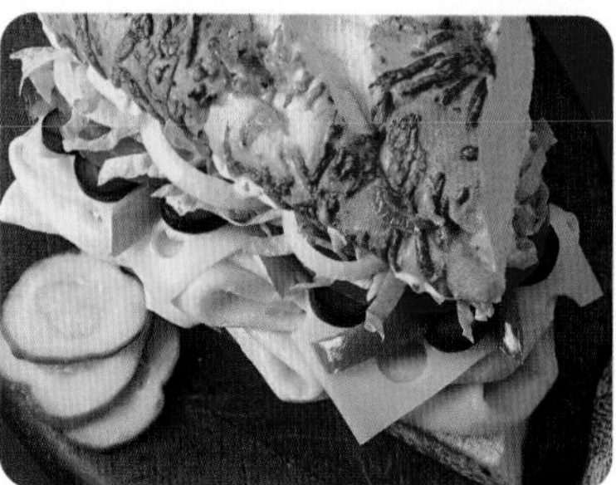

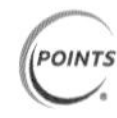

ColdSubs

BLIMPIE® Best® Sub (on white roll, with cheese, lettuce, tomato & onion), 6-inch 10

Club Sub (on white roll, with cheese, lettuce, tomato & onion), 6-inch 9

Ham & Cheese Sub (on white roll, with cheese, lettuce, tomato & onion), 6-inch 9

Roast Beef Sub (on white roll, with cheese, lettuce, tomato & onion), 6-inch 10

Seafood Sub (on white roll, without cheese, with lettuce, tomato & onion), 6-inch 7

Tuna Sub (on white roll, without cheese, with lettuce, tomato & onion), 6-inch 11

Turkey Sub (on white roll, with cheese, lettuce, tomato & onion), 6-inch 9

HotSubs

BLT Sub (on white roll, without cheese, with lettuce, tomato & onion), 6-inch 14

Grilled Chicken (on white roll, without cheese, with lettuce, tomato & onion), 6-inch 8

Buffalo Chicken (on white roll, with cheese, lettuce, tomato & onion), 6-inch 9

Meatball (on white roll, with cheese, lettuce, tomato & onion), 6-inch 13

Pastrami Sub (on white roll, with cheese, lettuce, tomato & onion), 6-inch 11

Steak & Onion (on white roll, with cheese, lettuce, tomato & onion), 6-inch 9

MexiMax™ (on white roll, without cheese, with lettuce, tomato & onion), 6-inch 8

ChikMax™ (on white roll, without cheese, with lettuce, tomato & onion), 6-inch 11

VegiMax™ (on white roll, without cheese, with lettuce, tomato & onion), 6-inch 8

GrilledSubs

Beef, Turkey & Cheddar, 6-inch 14

Cuban, 6-inch 10

Pastrami Special, 6-inch 10

Reuben, 6-inch 15

Ultimate Club, 6-inch 17

POINTS®

Wraps

Chicken Caesar Wrap, 6-inch 15
Beef & Cheddar Wrap, 6-inch 17
Southwestern Wrap, 6-inch 16
Steak & Onion Wrap, 6-inch 17
Ultimate BLT Wrap, 6-inch 20
Zesty Italian Wrap, 6-inch 15

Salads

Antipasto Salad, 1 regular serving 5
Chef Salad, 1 regular serving 4
Chicken Caesar Salad, 1 regular serving 9
Seafood Salad, 1 regular serving 2
Tuna Salad, 1 regular serving 6

SaladDressings

Bleu Cheese, 1.5 oz 7
BLIMPIE Dressing, 1.5 oz 5
Caesar, 1.5 oz 6
Dijon Honey Mustard, 1.5 oz 5
Fat Free Italian, 1.5 oz 1
Honey French, 1.5 oz 6
Light Ranch, 1.5 oz 2
Lite Italian, 1.5 oz 0
Parmesan Peppercorn, 1.5 oz 7
Pesto Dressing, 1 oz 4
Thousand Island, 1.5 oz 9

POINTS®

Extras

Cheddar Cheese, 1 slice 1
Provolone Cheese, 1 slice 2
Swiss Cheese, 1 slice 2
Oil & Vinegar Topping, 1 serving (for 6-inch sub) 1

Rolls

White, 6-inch 4
Wheat, 6-inch 4
Garden Italian Bread, 6-inch 5
Marbled Rye, 6-inch 6
Zesty Parmesan Bread, 6-inch 5
Honey Oat Bread, 6-inch 6
Wheat with Poppy Seed, 6-inch 4
Wheat with Sesame Seed, 6-inch 5
White with Poppy Seed, 6-inch 5
White with Sesame Seed, 6-inch 5
Flour Tortilla, 1 7
Spinach Tortilla, 1 6
Mediterranean Flat Bread, 1 6

Note: The nutritional information used for the above information is based on independent laboratory analysis and from data from our product suppliers and the U.S. Department of Agriculture. The nutritional information is derived from our standard product formulas.

Some Low-*POINT* Ideas

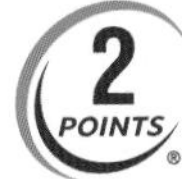

1 regular serving Seafood Salad

1 regular serving Chef Salad

1 regular serving Antipasto Salad

1 regular serving Tuna Salad

Bob Evans®

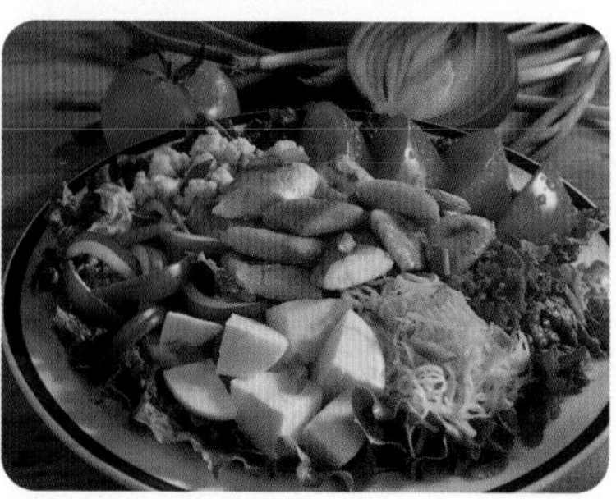

Salad (without roll)

Cobb Salad/Lunch Savor, 1 serving 13
Fruit Plate, 1 7
Garden Salad, without dressing, 1 4

SaladDressings

Fat-Free Ranch Dressing, 3 Tbsp 1
Lite Italian Dressing, 3 Tbsp 2

Soups

Bean Soup, 1 cup 3
Bean Soup, 1 bowl 4
Vegetable Soup, 1 cup 3
Vegetable Soup, 1 bowl 5

Entrees (without side dishes or roll)

Chicken & Noodles, 1 serving 9
Chicken Tender Marinated, 1 piece 2
Fried Cod, 1 serving 9
Grilled Chicken Sandwich, plain, 1 8
Ham Steak, 1 slice 2
Spaghetti with Marinara Sauce, 1 serving 13

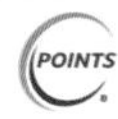

Stir-Fry, Vegetable, Lunch Savor, 1 serving (dinner portion) 7
Turkey & Dressing Dinner, 1 serving 15
Turkey, sliced, 1 serving 1

SideDishes&Bread

Apple Sauce, 1 serving 2
Baked Potato, Seasoned (plain), 1 serving 4
Bread & Celery Stuffing, 1 serving 5
Carrots Glazed, 1 serving 4
Cole Slaw, 1 serving 6
Cottage Cheese, 1 serving 3
Dinner Rolls, 2 plain 9
French Fries, 1 serving 5
Green Beans, 1 serving 2
Grilled Vegetables, 1 serving 2
Mashed Potatoes, 1 serving 4
Orange-Cranberry Relish, 1 serving 1
Rice Pilaf, 1 serving 5
Sourdough Bread, 1 slice 3

Breakfast

Bacon, 1 serving 1
Biscuit, 2 plain 10
Blueberry Hotcakes, plain, 1 4
Canadian Bacon, 1 serving 1
Egg Beaters®, 1 serving 3
French Toast, 1 serving (2 pieces) 6
Garden Harvest Omelette (made with Egg Beaters®), 1 serving 8
Grits (plain), 1 serving 4
Ham & Cheese Omelette (made with Egg Beaters®), 1 serving 8

Home Fries, 1 serving 3
Hot Chocolate, 1 serving 3
Hotcake, 1 plain 4
Lite Sausage Link, 1 3
Oatmeal, 1 serving 2
Sausage Link, 1 2
Sausage Patty, 1 4
Western Omelette (made with Egg Beaters®), 1 serving 8

Gravies

Beef Gravy, 1 serving 1
Chicken Gravy, 1 serving 2
Country Gravy, 1 serving 1
Sausage Gravy, 1 cup 6

MealIdeas

2 servings Sliced Turkey with 1 serving Orange-Cranberry Relish
1 serving Green Beans

1 slice Ham Steak
1 serving Grilled Vegetables
1 slice Sourdough Bread

1 serving Western or Ham & Cheese Omelette (made with Egg Beaters®)
1 serving Home Fries

Bojangles'®

POINTS

CajunSpiced™Chicken
Breast, 1 (as served with skin) ... 7
Leg, 1 (as served with skin) ... 6
Thigh, 1 (as served with skin) ... 8
Wing, 1 (as served with skin) ... 9

SouthernStyleChicken
Breast, 1 (as served with skin) ... 6
Leg, 1 (as served with skin) ... 6
Thigh, 1 (as served with skin) ... 8
Wing, 1 (as served with skin) ... 8

SweetBiscuits
Bo Berry® Biscuit, 1 ... 5
Cinnamon Biscuit, 1 ... 8

Biscuit&BiscuitSandwiches
Bacon Biscuit, 1 ... 7
Bacon, Egg & Cheese Biscuit, 1 ... 14
Biscuit, plain, 1 ... 5
Cajun Filet Biscuit, 1 ... 11
Country Ham Biscuit, 1 ... 6
Egg Biscuit, 1 ... 10
Sausage Biscuit, 1 ... 9
Smoked Sausage Biscuit, 1 ... 10
Steak Biscuit, 1 ... 17

Sandwiches
Cajun Filet Sandwich, with mayonnaise, 1 ... 10
Cajun Filet Sandwich, without mayonnaise, 1 ... 7

POINTS

Cajun Steak Sandwich, with horseradish sauce and pickles, 1 ... 10
Grilled Filet Sandwich, with mayonnaise, 1 ... 8
Grilled Filet Sandwich, without mayonnaise, 1 ... 5

IndividualFixin'
Bo Rounds®, 1 serving ... 6
Cajun Pintos®, 1 serving ... 2
Corn on the Cob, 1 serving ... 3
Dirty Rice®, 1 serving ... 4
Green Beans, 1 serving ... 1
Macaroni & Cheese, 1 serving ... 5
Marinated Cole Slaw, 1 serving ... 3
Potatoes, without gravy, 1 serving ... 2
Seasoned Fries, 1 serving ... 8

Snacks
Buffalo Bites, 1 serving ... 4
Chicken Supremes, 1 serving ... 8

MealIdeas

1 serving Cajun Pintos®
1 serving Potatoes (without gravy)
1 serving Green Beans

1 serving Buffalo Bites
1 serving Potatoes (without gravy)
1 serving Cajun Pintos®

1 Grilled Filet Sandwich (without mayonnaise)
1 serving Dirty Rice®

Boston Market®

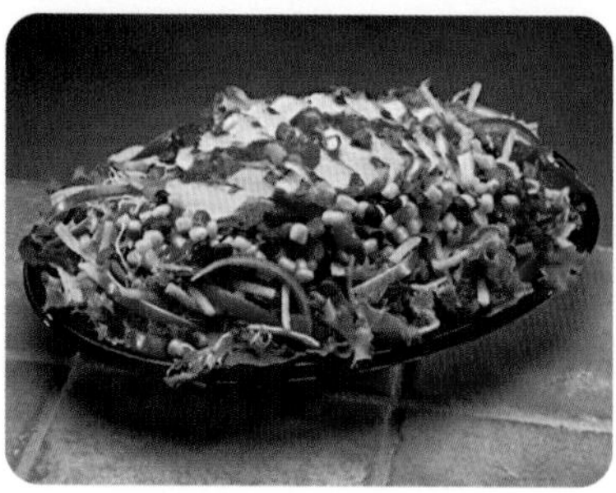

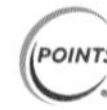

Entrees

Chicken, ½ (with skin) 15
Dark Meat Chicken, ¼ (served with skin) 8
Dark Meat Chicken, ¼ (skin removed by customer) 5
White Meat Chicken, ¼ (skin and wing removed by customer) 4
White Meat Chicken, ¼ (served with skin and wing) 7
Chunky Chicken Salad, 1 serving (¾ cup) 13
Chicken Pot Pie, 1 18
Grilled Chicken, BBQ, 1 9
Grilled Chicken, Teriyaki, 1 6
Honey Glazed Ham, 1 serving 5
Marinated Grilled Chicken, 1 5
Meat Loaf & Brown Gravy, 1 serving 9
Meat Loaf & Chunky Tomato Sauce, 1 serving 8
Meatloaf, 1 serving 8
Skinless Rotisserie Turkey Breast, 1 serving 3
Turkey Pot Pie, 1 17

Sandwiches

BBQ Chicken, shredded, 1 12
BBQ Grilled Chicken (no cheese or mayonnaise), 1 12
BBQ Grilled Chicken, 1 20
Chicken, with cheese and sauce, 1 14
Chicken, without cheese and sauce, 1 8
Ham, with cheese and sauce, 1 15
Ham, without cheese and sauce, 1 8
Marinated Grilled Chicken (no mayonnaise), 1 10
Marinated Grilled Chicken, 1 16
Meatloaf, with cheese, 1 16
Open Faced Meatloaf Sandwich, 1 meal 17
Open Faced Turkey Sandwich, 1 meal 15
Teriyaki Grilled Chicken, 1 15
Turkey Bacon Club, 1 18
Turkey, with cheese and sauce, 1 14
Turkey, without cheese and sauce, 1 8

Soups

Chicken Noodle Soup, 6 oz 2
Chicken Tortilla Soup (with toppings), ¾ cup 4
Chicken Tortilla Soup (no toppings), ¾ cup 2
Turkey Tortilla Soup (with toppings), ¾ cup 3
Turkey Tortilla Soup (no toppings), ¾ cup 1

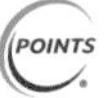

HotSideDishes

Butternut Squash, 1 serving (¾ cup)......3
Chicken Gravy, 2 Tbsp 0
Creamed Spinach, 1 serving (¾ cup)......6
Green Bean Casserole, 1 serving (¾ cup)......2
Green Beans, 1 serving (¾ cup)......2
Homestyle Mashed Potatoes & Gravy, 1 serving (¾ cup)......5
Homestyle Mashed Potatoes, 1 serving (⅔ cup)......5
Hot Cinnamon Apples, 1 serving (¾ cup)......5
Macaroni & Cheese, 1 serving (¾ cup) ...6
New Potatoes, 1 serving (¾ cup) 2
Rice Pilaf, 1 serving (⅔ cup) 3
Savory Stuffing, 1 serving (¾ cup) 4
Steamed Vegetables, 1 serving (⅔ cup)......0
Sweet Potato Casserole, 1 6
Whole Kernel Corn, 1 serving (¾ cup) 4

ColdSideDishes

Coleslaw, 1 serving (¾ cup) 7
Cranberry Walnut Relish, 1 serving (¾ cup)......7
Fruit Salad, 1 serving (¾ cup) 1
Jumpin Juice Squares, 1 serving 3
Old-Fashioned Potato Salad, 1 serving (¾ cup) 5
Tortellini Salad, 1 serving (¾ cup) 9

Salads

Caesar Salad Entree, with dressing, 1......17
Caesar Salad Entree, without dressing, 1 5
Caesar Side Salad (with dressing), 1....12
Chicken Caesar Salad (with dressing), 1......21
Oriental Grill Chicken Salad (no dressing or noodles), 1......6
Oriental Grill Chicken Salad (with dressing & noodles), 1 14
Southwest Grill Chicken Salad (no dressing or chips), 1 11
Southwest Grill Chicken Salad (with dressing & chips), 1 22

BakedGoods

Apple Struessel Pie, 1 slice......10
Cheesecake, 1 slice 15
Cherry Struesel Pie, 1 slice 8
Chocolate Cake, 1 slice 15
Cornbread, 1 loaf......4
Family Nestle® Brownie, 1 serving (¼ tray) 3
Hummingbird Cake, 1 slice 17
Nestle® Brownie, 1 13
Nestle® Toll House Peanut Butter Chip Cookie, 1 10
Nestle® Toll House Chocolate Chip Cookie, 1 9
Nestle® Toll House Oatmeal Scotchie Cookie, 1 9

Baked Goods (con't)

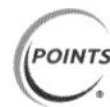

Oreo® Brownie with nestle chocolate chips, 1 19
Pecan Pie, 1 slice 12
Pumpkin Pie, 1 slice 6
Rice Krispie Treat, 1 bar 9

MealIdeas

¾ cup Turkey Tortilla Soup (without toppings)
1 serving Skinless Rotisserie Turkey Breast
1 serving Steamed Vegetables

6 oz Chicken Noodle Soup
¼ White Meat Chicken (without skin and wing) with 2 Tbsp Chicken Gravy
1 serving New Potatoes

1 Chicken, Ham, or Turkey Sandwich (without cheese and sauce)
1 serving Fruit Salad

Breadsmith®

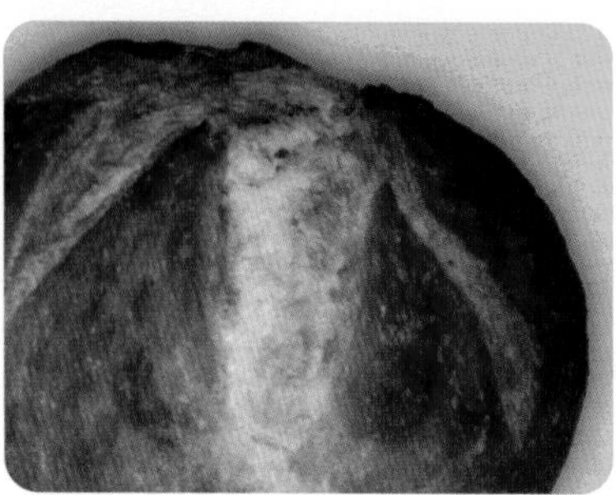

Item	POINTS
Apple Pie Bread, 1 oz	2
Austrian Pumpernickel, 1 oz	1
Banana Dessert Bread, 1 oz	2
Beer Bread, 1 oz	1
Blueberry Corn Dessert Bread, 1 oz	2
Blueberry Cornbread, 1 oz	1
Blueberry Lemon, 1 oz	1
Cheddar Sourdough, 1 oz	1
Cherry Walnut, 1 oz	1
Chocolate Bread, 1 oz	2
Chocolate Cherry Bread, 1 oz	2
Chocolate Chip Cookie, 1 oz	3
Chocolate Dessert Bread, 1 oz	2
Ciabatta, 1 oz	1
Cinnamon Spice, 1 oz	2
Country Buttertop, 1 oz	1
Cranberry Orange Dessert Bread, 1 oz	2
Dark Rye, 1 oz	1
English Muffin, 1 oz	1
Flax Seed, 1 oz	1
Focaccia, 1 oz	1
Freedom Bread, 1 oz	2

Item	POINTS
French Peasant, 1 oz	1
French, 1 oz	1
Fruit Bread, 1 oz	1
Garlic Onion Parmesan, 1 oz	1
Garlic Onion, 1 oz	1
Gluten Free, 1 oz	2
Greek Olive, 1 oz	1
Hamburger Buns, 1 oz	2
Honey Oat Bran, 1 oz	1
Honey Raisin, 1 oz	1
Honey Sunflower Whole Wheat, 1 oz	1
Honey Wheat, 1 oz	1
Honey White, 1 oz	1
Honey Whole Wheat, 1 oz	1
Hot Cross Buns, 1 oz	2
Irish Oat Bran, 1 oz	1
Irish Soda Bread, 1 oz	2
Jalapeno Cornbread, 1 oz	1
Light Rye, 1 oz	1
Maple Walnut, 1 oz	2
Marathon Multigrain, 1 oz	1
Mediterranean Herb, 1 oz	1
Multigrain Light with Rosemary, 1 oz	1
Multigrain, 1 oz	1
Norwegian Rye, 1 oz	1
Onion Rye, 1 oz	1
Peppercorn Swiss, 1 oz	2
Pepperoni Bread, 1 oz	2
Pesto, 1 oz	1
Pizza Dough, 1 oz	2
Potato Cheddar Chive, 1 oz	1
Pumpkin Dessert Bread, 1 oz	2
Raisin Cinnamon Walnut, 1 oz	1

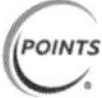

Item	POINTS
Raisin Cinnamon, 1 oz	1
Raisin Sunflower, 1 oz	1
Raisin Walnut, 1 oz	1
Rosemary Fougasse, 1 oz	1
Rosemary Garlic Ciabatta, 1 oz	1
Rustic Italian, 1 oz	1
Sourdough Rye, 1 oz	1
Sourdough, 1 oz	1
Stoneground Wheat, 1 oz	1
Sweet Bellagio, 1 oz	1
Tomato Basil, 1 oz	1
Traditional Rye, 1 oz	1
Tuscan Herb Formaggio, 1 oz	1
Tuscan Rustica, 1 oz	1
Vanilla Egg, 1 oz	2

Some Low-*POINT* Ideas

each

1 oz each
- Austrian Pumpernickel
- Country Buttertop
- Garlic Onion Parmesan
- Pesto
- Sourdough Rye

each

Dessert Breads (1 oz each)
- Banana
- Blueberry Corn
- Chocolate
- Cranberry Orange
- Pumpkin

BRUEGGER'S BAGELS®

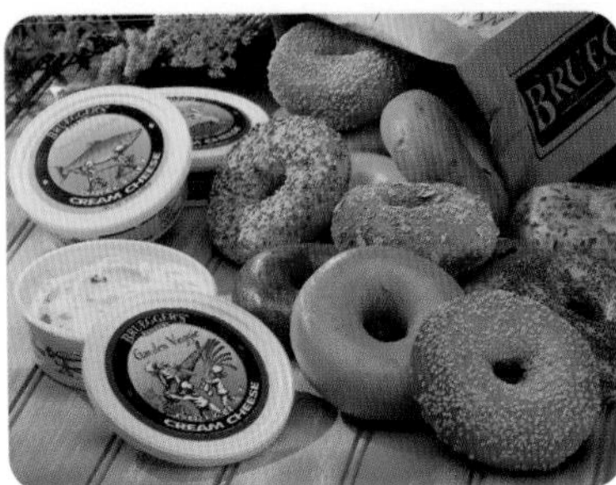

POINTS

Bagels (without spread)

- **Banana Nut Bagel,** 1 7
- **Blueberry Bagel,** 1 6
- **Chocolate Chip Bagel,** 1 5
- **Cinnamon Raisin Bagel,** 1 5
- **Cranberry Orange Bagel,** 1 5
- **Egg Bagel,** 1 6
- **Everything Bagel,** 1 5
- **Garlic Bagel,** 1 5
- **Honey Grain Bagel,** 1 6
- **Jalapeño Bagel,** 1 5
- **Onion Bagel,** 1 6
- **Plain Bagel,** 1 6
- **Poppy Bagel,** 1 6
- **Pumpernickel Bagel,** 1 5
- **Rosemary Olive Oil Bagel,** 1 6
- **Salt Bagel,** 1 6
- **Sesame Bagel,** 1 6
- **Sourdough Bagel,** 1 5
- **Spinach Herb Bagel,** 1 5
- **Sundried Tomato Bagel,** 1 5

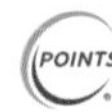

Bruegger's® Cream Cheese and Hummus

- **Bruegger's® Plain Cream Cheese,** 3 Tbsp 4
- **Bruegger's® Bacon Scallion Cream Cheese,** 3 Tbsp 4
- **Bruegger's® Chive Cream Cheese,** 3 Tbsp 4
- **Bruegger's® Cucumber Dill Cream Cheese,** 3 Tbsp 4
- **Bruegger's® Garden Veggie Cream Cheese,** 3 Tbsp 4
- **Bruegger's® Honey Walnut Cream Cheese,** 3 Tbsp 4
- **Bruegger's® Jalapeño Cream Cheese,** 3 Tbsp 4
- **Bruegger's® Light Garden Veggie Cream Cheese,** 3 Tbsp 2
- **Bruegger's® Light Plain Cream Cheese,** 3 Tbsp 2
- **Bruegger's® Light Strawberry Cream Cheese,** 3 Tbsp 2
- **Bruegger's® Olive Pimento Cream Cheese,** 3 Tbsp 4
- **Bruegger's® Salmon Cream Cheese,** 3 Tbsp 4
- **Bruegger's® Wildberry Cream Cheese,** 3 Tbsp 4
- **Hummus,** 2 Tbsp 1

Deli-Style Bagel Sandwiches

- **Chicken Salad Sandwich,** 1 9
- **Deli-Style Ham Sandwich, with lettuce, tomato, and mustard,** 1 11

POINTS

Deli-Style Turkey Sandwich, with lettuce, tomato, and mustard, 1 .... **10**
Garden Veggie Sandwich (Swiss cheese, lettuce, tomato, alfalfa sprouts, cucumber slices, and mustard), 1 .... **9**
Hummus Sandwich, 1 .... **10**
Tuna Salad Sandwich, 1 .... **11**

Specialty Bagel Sandwiches

Chicken Fajita, 1 .... **11**
Herby Turkey®, 1 .... **12**
Leonardo Da Veggie®, 1 .... **10**
Santa Fe Turkey, 1 .... **10**

Bagel & Egg Sandwiches

Egg and Cheese Sandwich, 1 .... **10**
Egg and Sausage Sandwich, 1 .... **14**
Egg Sandwich, 1 .... **8**
Egg, Ham and Cheese Sandwich, 1 .... **11**

Soups & Stew

Aztec Chicken Soup, 1 cup **2**
Aztec Chicken Soup, 1 bowl **3**
Chicken Noodle Soup, 1 cup **3**
Chicken Noodle Soup, 1 bowl **4**
Garden Split Pea Soup, 1 cup **3**
Garden Split Pea Soup, 1 bowl **4**
Marcello Minestrone Soup, 1 cup **1**
Marcello Minestrone Soup, 1 bowl **1**
New England Clam Chowder, 1 cup **4**
New England Clam Chowder, 1 bowl **6**
Ratatouille Stew, 1 cup **1**

POINTS

Ratatouille Stew, 1 bowl **1**
Terrific Turkey Orzo Soup, 1 cup **2**
Terrific Turkey Orzo Soup, 1 bowl **2**

Desserts

Bruegger Bar, 1 .... **10**
Luscious Lemon Bars, 1 .... **9**
Pecan Chocolate Chunk, 1 .... **9**
Raspberry Sammies, 1 .... **7**

Meal Ideas

1 bowl Ratatouille Stew
1 Spinach Herb Bagel (without spread)

1 Everything Bagel with 3 Tbsp Bruegger's® Light Garden Veggie Cream Cheese

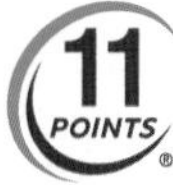

1 Hummus Deli-Style Bagel Sandwich
1 bowl Marcello Minestrone Soup

BURGER KING®

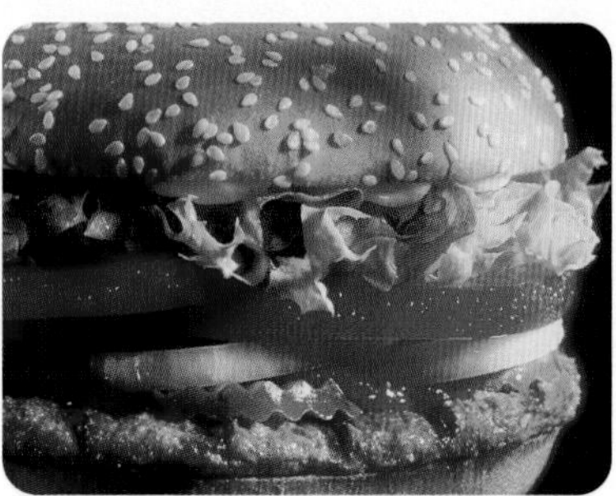

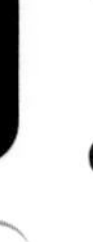

Burgers&Sandwiches

Hamburger, 1 7
Cheeseburger, 1 8
Double Hamburger, 1 11
Double Cheeseburger, 1 13
Bacon Double Cheeseburger, 1 14
BK FISH FILET™ Sandwich, 1 13
BK VEGGIE™ Burger, 1 7
BK VEGGIE™ Burger, without reduced fat mayonnaise, 1 6
Chicken WHOPPER JR.®, 1 8
Chicken WHOPPER JR.®, without mayonnaise, 1 6
Chicken WHOPPER®, 1 13
Chicken WHOPPER®, without mayonnaise, 1 9
KING SUPREME™ Sandwich, 1 13
Original DOUBLE WHOPPER® Sandwich, 1 26

POINTS

Original DOUBLE WHOPPER® Sandwich, without mayonnaise, 1 21
Original DOUBLE WHOPPER® with Cheese Sandwich, 1 29
Original DOUBLE WHOPPER® with Cheese Sandwich, without mayonnaise, 1 24
Original WHOPPER JR.® Sandwich, 1 9
Original WHOPPER JR.® Sandwich, without mayonnaise, 1 7
Original WHOPPER JR.® with Cheese Sandwich, 1 11
Original WHOPPER JR.® with Cheese Sandwich, without mayonnaise, 1 8
Original WHOPPER® Sandwich, 1 18
Original WHOPPER® Sandwich, without mayonnaise, 1 14
Original WHOPPER® with Cheese Sandwich, 1 21
Original WHOPPER® with Cheese Sandwich, without mayonnaise, 1 16
Specialty Chicken Sandwich, 1 13
Specialty Chicken Sandwich, without mayonnaise, 1 10

CHICKENTENDERS®&Sauces

CHICKEN TENDERS®, 4 pieces 4
CHICKEN TENDERS®, 5 pieces 5
CHICKEN TENDERS®, 6 pieces 6
CHICKEN TENDERS®, 8 pieces 8
Barbecue Dipping Sauce, 1 packet (2 Tbsp) 1
Honey Flavored Dipping Sauce, 1 packet (2 Tbsp) 2
Honey Mustard Dipping Sauce, 1 packet (2 Tbsp) 2
Ranch Dipping Sauce, 1 packet (2 Tbsp) 4
Sweet & Sour Dipping Sauce, 1 packet (2 Tbsp) 1

SideOrders

French Fries (salted), 1 small serving 5
French Fries (salted), 1 medium serving 8
French Fries (salted), 1 large serving 11
French Fries (salted), 1 king size serving 14
Onion Rings, 1 small serving 4
Onion Rings, 1 medium serving 7
Onion Rings, 1 large serving 11
Onion Rings, 1 king size serving 12

Salads

Chicken Caesar (without dressing and croutons), 1 3
Garden Salad (without dressing), 1 0

SaladDressings

KRAFT® Catalina Dressing, 1 serving (43 g) 5
KRAFT® Fat Free Ranch Dressing, 1 serving (43 g) 1
KRAFT® Ranch Dressing, 1 serving (43 g) 6
KRAFT® Thousand Island Dressing, 1 serving (43 g) 3
LIGHT DONE RIGHT® Lite Italian Dressing, 1 serving (43 g) 1
SIGNATURE® Creamy Caesar Dressing, 1 serving (43 g) 4

Breakfast

Breakfast Syrup, 1 packet (2 Tbsp) 2
CROISSAN'WICH® with Sausage and Cheese, 1 11
CROISSAN'WICH® with Egg & Cheese, 1 8
CROISSAN'WICH® with Sausage, Egg, and Cheese, 1 13
SOURDOUGH Breakfast Sandwich with Bacon, Egg & Cheese, 1 9
SOURDOUGH Breakfast Sandwich with Ham, Egg & Cheese, 1 9
SOURDOUGH Breakfast Sandwich with Sausage, Egg & Cheese, 1 14
French Toast Sticks, without syrup, 5 sticks 9
Hash Brown Rounds, 1 small serving 5
Hash Brown Rounds, 1 large serving 9
Grape or Strawberry Jam, 1 packet (2 Tbsp) 1

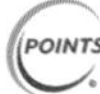

Shakes, Frozen Beverages & Dessert

Chocolate Shake, syrup added, 1 small 15
Chocolate Shake, syrup added, 1 medium 19
Vanilla Shake, 1 small 14
Vanilla Shake, 1 medium 18
Strawberry Shake, syrup added, 1 small 15
Strawberry Shake, syrup added, 1 small 19
Dutch Apple Pie, 1 serving 8
Fresh Baked Cookies, 1 10
Frozen COCA COLA® Classic, 1 medium 7
Frozen COCA COLA® Classic, 1 large 9
Frozen MINUTE MAID® Cherry, 1 medium 7
Frozen MINUTE MAID® Cherry, 1 large 9
HERSHEY'S® Sundae Pie, 1 serving 8

Meal Ideas

4 pieces CHICKEN TENDERS® with
1 packet Barbecue Dipping Sauce
1 Garden Salad with
1 serving KRAFT® Fat Free Ranch Dressing

4 pieces CHICKEN TENDERS® with
1 packet Sweet & Sour Dipping Sauce
1 small serving Onion Rings

1 Chicken WHOPPER JR.® (without mayonnaise)
1 small serving Onion Rings
1 Garden Salad with
1 serving LIGHT DONE RIGHT® Lite Italian Dressing

Carl's Jr.®

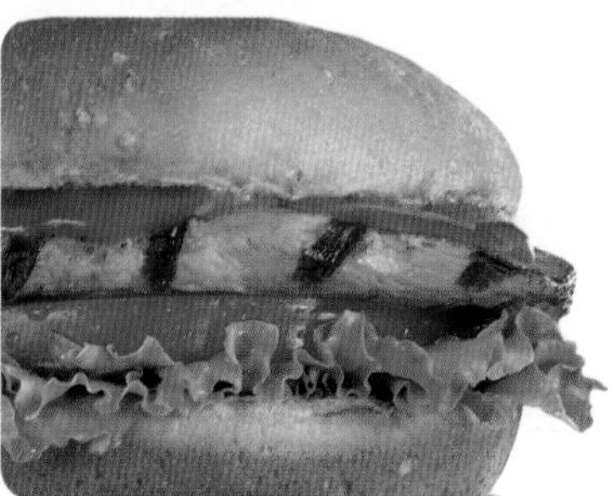

POINTS

Burgers&Sandwiches

Hamburger, 1 6
Carl's Famous Star® Hamburger, 1 14
Super Star® Hamburger, 1 19
Famous Bacon Cheeseburger, 1 17
Sourdough Bacon Cheeseburger, 1 16
Sourdough Ranch Bacon Cheeseburger, 1 18
Western Bacon Cheeseburger®, 1 15
Double Western Bacon Cheeseburger®, 1 22
Double Sourdough Bacon Cheeseburger, 1 22
Spicy Chicken Sandwich, 1 11
Southwest Spicy Chicken Sandwich, 1 15
Carl's Ranch Crispy Chicken Sandwich, 1 15
Carl's Bacon Swiss Crispy Chicken Sandwich, 1 18
Carl's Western Bacon Crispy Chicken Sandwich, 1 17
Charbroiled BBQ Chicken Sandwich™, 1 6

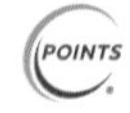

Charbroiled BBQ Club Sandwich™, 1 11
Charbroiled Santa Fe Chicken Sandwich™, 1 13
Charbroiled Sirloin Steak Sandwich, 1 13
Carl's Catch Fish Sandwich™, 1 13

GreatStuff™Potatoes

Plain Potato, without margarine, 1 5
Bacon & Cheese Potato, 1 14
Broccoli & Cheese Potato, 1 12
Sour Cream & Chives Potato, 1 9

Salads&SaladDressings

Charbroiled Chicken Salad-To-Go™, without dressing, 1 4
Garden Salad-To-Go™, without dressing, 1 1
Blue Cheese Dressing, 1 packet (approx. 4 Tbsp) 9
Fat-Free French Dressing, 1 packet (approx. 4 Tbsp) 1
Fat-Free Italian Dressing, 1 packet (approx. 4 Tbsp) 0
House Dressing, 1 packet (approx. 4 Tbsp) 6
Thousand Island Dressing, 1 packet (approx. 4 Tbsp) 7

SideOrders

Chicken Stars, 6 pieces 6
CrissCut Fries®, 1 serving 9
French Fries, 1 kid's serving 6
French Fries, 1 small serving 6

POINTS

French Fries, 1 medium serving 10
French Fries, 1 large serving 14
Onion Rings, 1 serving 10
Zucchini, 1 serving 8

Sauces

BBQ Sauce, 1 packet (2 Tbsp) 1
Honey Sauce, 1 packet (2 Tbsp) 2
Mustard Sauce, 1 packet (2 Tbsp) 1
Sweet N' Sour Sauce, 1 packet (2 Tbsp) 1

Breakfast

Breakfast Burrito, 1 13
Breakfast Quesadilla, 1 9
Sunrise Sandwich®, without bacon or sausage, 1 9
Sourdough Breakfast, 1 10
French Toast Dips®, without syrup, 1 serving 9
Table Syrup, 1 packet (2 Tbsp) 2
Scrambled Eggs, 1 serving 5
English Muffin with Margarine, 1 5
Bacon, 2 pieces 1
Sausage, 1 patty 5
Hash Brown Nuggets, 1 serving 8

Bakery Items & Desserts

Cheese Danish, 1 10
Blueberry Muffin, 1 8
Bran Raisin Muffin, 1 8
Chocolate Cake, 1 serving 7
Strawberry Swirl Cheesecake, 1 serving 7
Chocolate Chip Cookie, 1 serving 8

POINTS

Shakes

Chocolate Shake, 1 small 11
Chocolate Shake, 1 regular 16
Strawberry Shake, 1 small 11
Strawberry Shake, 1 regular 16
Vanilla Shake, 1 small 10
Vanilla Shake, 1 regular 15

Meal Ideas

1 Charbroiled Chicken Salad-To-Go™ with 1 packet Fat-Free Italian Dressing

1 Hamburger
1 Garden Salad-To-Go™ with 1 packet Fat-Free French Dressing

1 Breakfast Quesadilla
2 pieces Bacon

Carvel® Ice Cream Bakery

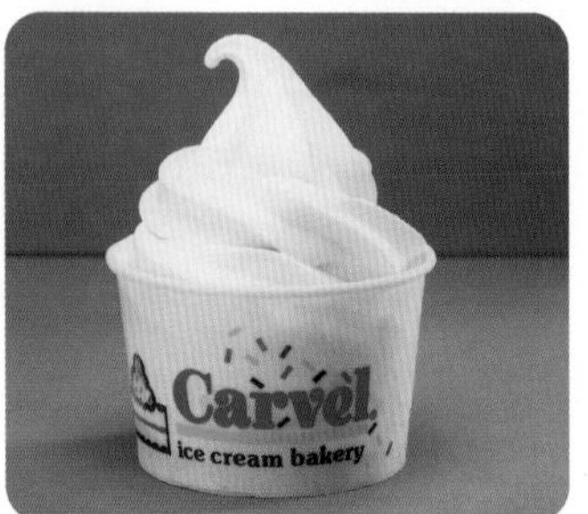

IceCream&Sherbet

Carvel Chocolate Ice Cream Cone, 1 regular cone 6

Carvel Chocolate Ice Cream, 1 regular serving 5

Carvel No Fat Chocolate Ice Cream, 1 regular serving 3

Carvel No Fat Vanilla Ice Cream, 1 regular serving 3

Carvel Sherbet (any flavor), 1 regular serving 3

Carvel Vanilla Ice Cream Cone, 1 regular cone 7

Carvel Vanilla Ice Cream, 1 regular serving 6

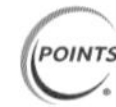

MilkShakes&SherbetFizzlers®

No Fat Chocolate Milk Shake, 1 regular serving 10

No Fat Chocolate Milk Shake, 1 small serving 7

No Fat Vanilla Milk Shake, 1 regular serving 8

No Fat Vanilla Milk Shake, 1 small serving 6

Sherbet Fizzlers®, 1 regular serving 7

Thick Chocolate Shake, 1 regular serving 17

Thick Vanilla Shake, 1 regular serving 15

NoveltyItems (from the freezer case)

Brown Bonnet® Cone, 1 9

Carvel No Fat Cone, 1 4

Chipsters Sandwich, 1 8

Flying Saucer®, chocolate, 1 5

Flying Saucer®, vanilla, 1 5

Piece of Cake, Cookies 'N Cream, 1 serving 6

Piece of Cake, Original, 1 serving 6

Piece of Cake, Sinfully Chocolate, 1 serving 7

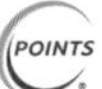

Cakes

Butterscotch Dream Ice Cream Cake, 1 slice (1/8 cake) 6

Carvel Small Round Cake, 1 slice (1/15 cake) 5

Cookies & Cream Ice Cream Cake, 1 slice (1/8 cake) 6

Crunch 'N Fudge Cake, 1(1/15 of cake) 6

Fudge Drizzle Ice Cream Cake, 1 slice (1/8 cake) 6

Fudgie The Whale Cake, 1 slice (1/12 of cake) 7

Large Sheet Cake, 1 slice (1/26 of large sheet cake) 5

Low Fat Cake, 1 slice (1/15 of 10" cake) 4

Sinfully Chocolate Ice Cream Cake, 1 slice (1/8 cake) 5

Small Sheet Cake, 1 slice (1/20 of small sheet cake) 6

Strawberries and Cream Ice Cream Cake, 1 slice (1/8 cake) 6

Some Low-*POINT* Ideas

each

1 regular serving Carvel No Fat Chocolate Ice Cream
1 regular serving Carvel No Fat Vanilla Ice Cream
1 regular serving Carvel Sherbet (any flavor)

each

1 Carvel No Fat Cone (from the freezer case)
1 slice Low Fat Cake

each

1 regular serving Carvel Chocolate Ice Cream
1 Chocolate or Vanilla Flying Saucer
1 slice Carvel Small Round Cake
1 slice Sinfully Chocolate Ice Cream Cake

Chick-fil-A®

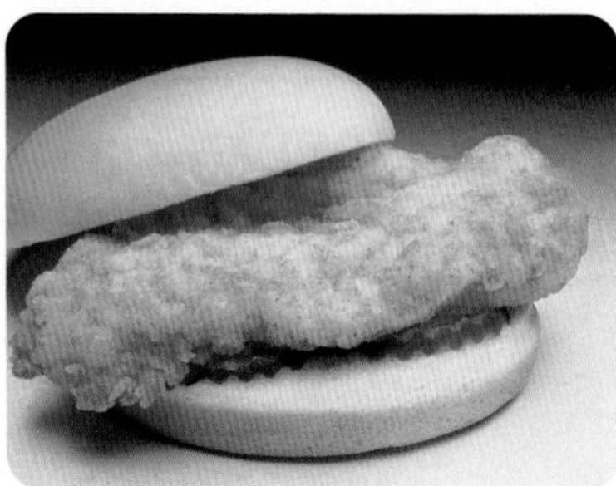

POINTS

Specialties

Chick-fil-A® Chicken Sandwich, 1 ... 9

Chick-fil-A® Chicken Sandwich (no butter), 1 ... 8

Chick-fil-A® Chicken Deluxe Sandwich, 1 ... 9

Chick-fil-A® Chargrilled Chicken Sandwich, 1 ... 6

Chick-fil-A® Chargrilled Chicken Sandwich (no butter), 1 ... 5

Chick-fil-A® Chargrilled Chicken Deluxe Sandwich, 1 ... 6

Chick-fil-A® Chargrilled Chicken Club Sandwich (no sauce), 1 ... 8

Chick-fil-A® Chick-n-Strips®, 4 pieces ... 6

Chick-fil-A® Nuggets, 8 pieces ... 6

Chick-fil-A® Chicken Salad Sandwich (on whole wheat bread), 1 ... 7

Chick-fil-A® Hearty Breast of Chicken Soup, 1 cup ... 3

POINTS

Chick-fil-A® Chargrilled Chicken Caesar Salad, without dressing, 1 ... 5

Chick-fil-A® Chargrilled Chicken Garden Salad, without dressing, 1 ... 4

Chick-fil-A® Chick-n-Strips® Salad, without dressing, 1 ... 8

Chick-fil-A® Chargrilled Chicken (no bun, no pickles), 1 fillet ... 2

Chick-fil-A® Chicken (no bun, no pickles), 1 fillet ... 6

Chick-fil-A® Chargrilled Chicken Cool Wrap®, 1 wrap ... 8

Chick-fil-A® Chicken Caesar Cool Wrap®, 1 wrap ... 10

Chick-fil-A® Spicy Chicken Cool Wrap®, 1 wrap ... 8

SideOrders

Carrot & Raisin Salad, 1 small serving ... 3

Waffle Potato Fries™, 1 small serving ... 6

Cole Slaw, 1 small serving ... 5

Side Salad, without dressing, 1 ... 2

DippingSauces

Barbecue Sauce, 1 packet ... 1

Dijon Honey Mustard Sauce, 1 packet ... 1

Honey Mustard Sauce, 1 packet ... 1

Polynesian Sauce, 1 packet ... 3

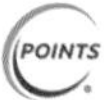

Croutons/Kernels

Garlic and Butter Croutons, 1 packet 2
Roasted Sunflower Kernels, 1 packet 2

SaladDressings

Basil Vinaigrette Dressing, 1 packet 6
Blue Cheese Dressing, 1 packet 5
Buttermilk Ranch Dressing, 1 packet 5
Caesar Dressing, 1 packet 6
Fat Free Dijon Honey Mustard Dressing, 1 packet 1
Light Italian Dressing, 1 packet 0
Spicy Dressing, 1 packet 6
Thousand Island Dressing, 1 packet 5

Desserts

Cheesecake, 1 slice 8
Cheesecake with Blueberry Topping, 1 slice 9
Cheesecake, with strawberry topping, 1 slice 9
Fudge Nut Brownie, 1 serving 8
Icedream®, 1 small cone 4
Icedream®, 1 small cup 5
Lemon Pie, 1 slice 7

MealIdeas

1 Chick-fil-A® Chargrilled Chicken Garden Salad with
1 packet Light Italian Dressing
1 small Icedream® Cone

1 Chick-fil-A® Chicken Salad Sandwich (on whole wheat bread)
1 Side Salad with
1 packet Fat-Free Dijon Honey Mustard Dressing

1 Chick-fil-A® Chargrilled Chicken Cool Wrap®
1 small serving Carrot & Raisin Salad

Churchs Chicken®

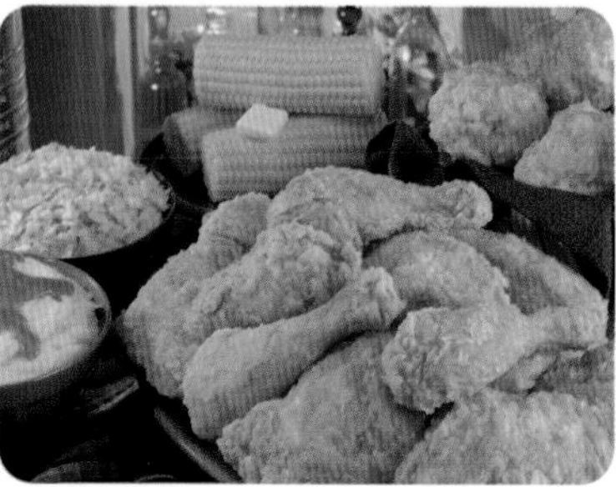

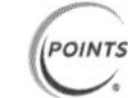

Fried Chicken

Breast, 1 (as served with skin) 5
Leg, 1 (as served with skin) 4
Thigh, 1 (as served with skin) 6
Wing, 1 (as served with skin) 6
Krispy Tender Strip™, 1 strip 3

CountryFriedSteak

Country Fried Steak with White Gravy, 1 serving (1 piece with gravy) 12

Sauces

BBQ Sauce, 1 package 1
Creamy Jalapeno Sauce, 1 package 3
Honey Mustard Sauce, 1 package 3
Purple Pepper Sauce™, 1 package 1
Sweet & Sour Sauce, 1 package 1

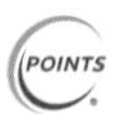

SideDishes&Dessert

Cajun Rice, 1 regular 3
Cole Slaw, 1 regular 2
Collard Greens, 1 regular 0
Corn on the Cob, 1 serving 2
French Fries, 1 regular 5
Honey Butter Biscuit, 1 (plain) 6
Jalapeño Cheese Bombers®, 4 5
Macaroni & Cheese, 1 regular 5
Okra, 1 regular 5
Potatoes & Gravy, 1 regular 2
Sweet Corn Nuggets, 1 regular 6
Tender Crunchers™, 1 serving (6-8 pieces) 9
Whole Jalapeño Peppers, 2 0
Apple Pie, 1 serving 6
Edward's Double Lemon Pie, 1 7
Edward's Strawberry Cream Cheese Pie, 1 6

Meal Ideas

1 Krispy Tender Strip
1 serving Corn on the Cob
1 regular Potatoes & Gravy

1 Fried Chicken Leg (with skin)
1 regular Cole Slaw
1 regular Cajun Rice

1 Fried Chicken Breast (with skin)
1 serving Corn on the Cob
1 regular Cajun Rice

Cousins Subs®

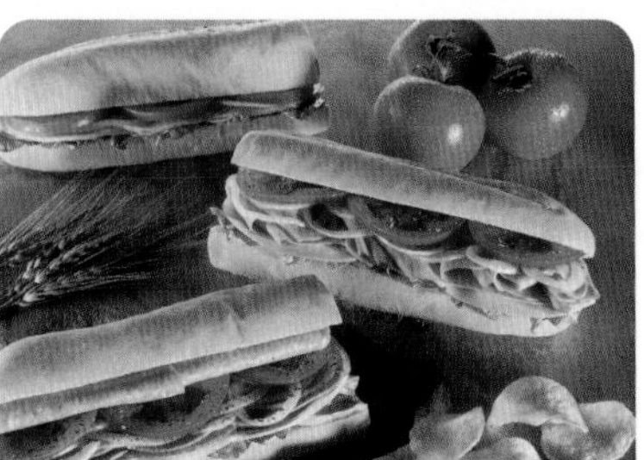

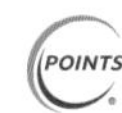

SubSandwiches (without mayonnaise and cheese, and no added salt)

BLT, ½ sub (7½" sub) 8
Chicken Breast, ½ sub (7½" sub) 8
Club, no cheese, ½ sub (7½" sub) 8
Cold Veggie, ½ sub (7½" sub) 5
Ham, ½ sub (7½" sub) 6
Hot Veggie, ½ sub (7½" sub) 6
Mini Ham, 1 4
Mini Turkey Breast, 1 4
Roast Beef, ½ sub (7½" sub) 7
Steak, ½ sub (7½" sub) 9
Turkey Breast, ½ sub (7½" sub) 6

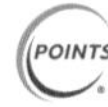

Soups

Chicken Noodle Soup, 1 regular 2
Chicken Noodle Soup, 1 large 4
Red Beans & Rice Soup, 1 regular 2
Red Beans & Rice Soup, 1 large 3
Tomato Basil Soup with Raviolini, 1 regular 2
Tomato Basil Soup with Raviolini, 1 large 3
Vegetable Beef Soup, 1 regular 2
Vegetable Beef Soup, 1 large 3

MealIdeas

1 regular Red Beans & Rice Soup
1 Mini Ham or Mini Turkey Breast Sub Sandwich (without mayonnaise and cheese)

1 regular Vegetable Beef Soup
½ Cold Veggie Sub Sandwich (without mayonnaise and cheese)

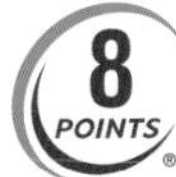

1 regular Chicken Noodle Soup
½ Turkey Breast, Ham, or Hot Veggie Sub Sandwich (without mayonnaise and cheese)

Dairy Queen® (United States)

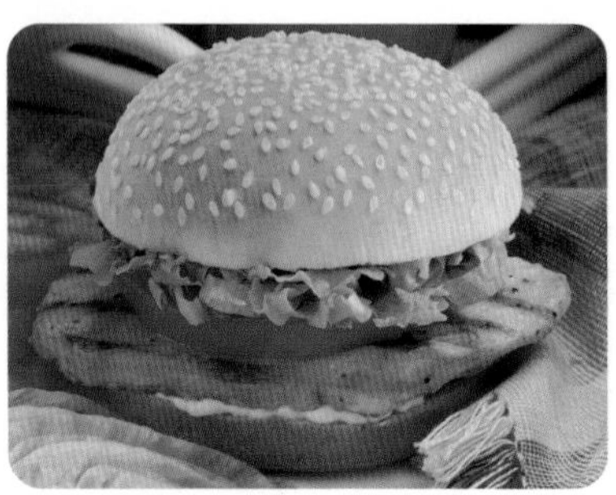

POINTS

SoftServeCones

Chocolate Cone, 1 small ... 5
Chocolate Cone, 1 medium ... 8
Dipped Cone, 1 small ... 8
Dipped Cone, 1 medium ... 12
DQ® Chocolate Soft Serve, ½ cup ... 3
DQ® Vanilla Soft Serve, ½ cup ... 3
Vanilla Cone, 1 small ... 5
Vanilla Cone, 1 medium ... 7
Vanilla Cone, 1 large ... 9

Sundaes

Chocolate Sundae, 1 small ... 6
Chocolate Sundae, 1 medium ... 9

RoyalTreats®

Banana Split, 1 ... 11
Brownie Earthquake®, 1 ... 17
Peanut Buster® Parfait, 1 ... 17
Pecan Mudslide™ Treat, 1 ... 15
Strawberry Shortcake, 1 ... 10

Novelties

Buster Bar®, 1 ... 11
Chocolate Dilly® Bar, 1 ... 5

POINTS

DQ® Fudge Bar, no sugar added, 1 ... 1
DQ® Sandwich, 1 ... 4
DQ® Vanilla Orange Bar, no sugar added, 1 ... 1
Lemon DQ Freez'r®, ½ cup ... 2
Starkiss®, 1 ... 2

Shakes,Malts,Misty®Slushes, &Smoothy

Chocolate Malt, 1 small ... 14
Chocolate Malt, 1 medium ... 19
Chocolate Shake, 1 small ... 12
Chocolate Shake, 1 medium ... 17
Frozen Hot Chocolate, 1 ... 20
Misty® Slush, 1 small ... 4
Misty® Slush, 1 medium ... 6

Blizzard®FlavorTreats

Chocolate Chip Cookie Dough Blizzard® Flavor Treat, 1 small ... 15
Chocolate Chip Cookie Dough Blizzard® Flavor Treat, 1 medium ... 22
Chocolate Sandwich Cookie Blizzard® Flavor Treat, 1 small ... 12
Chocolate Sandwich Cookie Blizzard® Flavor Treat, 1 medium ... 15

DQTreatzzaPizza®andCake

DQ® Frozen 8" Round Cake (undecorated), 1 slice (⅛ of cake) ... 8
DQ® Layered 8" Round Cake (undecorated), 1 slice (⅛ of cake) ... 8
Heath® DQ Treatzza Pizza®, 1 slice (⅛ of pizza) ... 4
M&M's® DQ Treatzza Pizza®, 1 slice (⅛ of pizza) ... 4

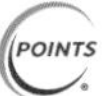

Brazier® Foods Only at Dairy Queen®/Brazier® Stores

DQ Homestyle® Hamburger, 1 6
DQ Homestyle® Cheeseburger, 1 8
DQ Homestyle® Double Cheeseburger, 1 13
DQ Homestyle® Bacon Double Cheeseburger, 1 15
DQ Ultimate® Burger, 1 17
Hot Dog, 1 6
Chili 'n' Cheese Dog, 1 8
Chicken Breast Fillet Sandwich, 1 11
Grilled Chicken Sandwich, 1 6
Chicken Strip Basket™ (4 breaded chicken strips, small French fries, Texas toast, and gravy), 1 23
French Fries, 1 small serving 8
French Fries, 1 medium serving 10
Onion Rings, 1 serving 7
Crispy Chicken™ Salad (with Fat Free Italian Dressing), 1 serving 11
Crispy Chicken™ Salad (with Honey Mustard Dressing), 1 serving 17
Grilled Chicken Salad (with Fat Free Italian Dressing), 1 serving 5
Grilled Chicken Salad (with Honey Mustard Dressing), 1 serving 11

Some Low-*POINT* Ideas

each

1 DQ® Fudge Bar (no sugar added)
1 DQ® Vanilla Orange Bar (no sugar added)

each

½ cup Lemon DQ Freez'r®
1 Starkiss®

Only at Dairy Queen®/ Brazier® Stores

1 serving Grilled Chicken Salad (with Fat Free Italian Dressing)

each

1 Grilled Chicken Sandwich
1 DQ Homestyle® Hamburger
1 Hot Dog

Dairy Queen® (Canada)

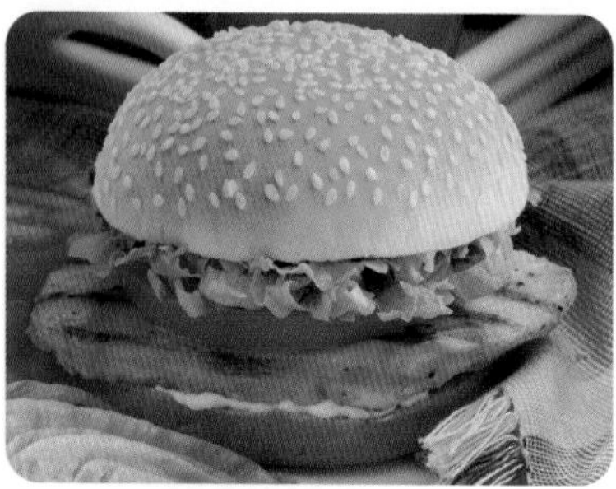

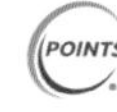

Cones

Chocolate Dipped Cone, 1 small 8
Chocolate Dipped Cone, 1 medium 11
DQ® Chocolate Soft Serve, ½ cup 4
DQ® Vanilla Soft Serve, ½ cup 4
Vanilla Cone, 1 small 5
Vanilla Cone, 1 medium 7

Blizzard® Flavour Treats

Oreo® Blizzard®, 1 small 13
Oreo® Blizzard®, 1 medium 16
Skor® Blizzard®, 1 small 14
Skor® Blizzard®, 1 medium 22

Royal Treats®

Banana Split, 1 serving 15
Peanut Buster® Parfait, 1 serving 17
Pecan Mudslide™, 1 serving 15

POINTS

Novelties

Buster Bar®, 1 12
Dilly® Bar, 1 5
DQ® Sandwich, 1 3

Misty® Slushes

Berry Cherry Smoothy, 1 16
Cherry Misty® Slush, 1 small 7
Cherry Misty® Slush, 1 medium 11

Sundaes

Cherry Sundae, 1 small 6
Cherry Sundae, 1 medium 9
Chocolate Sundae, 1 small 7
Chocolate Sundae, 1 medium 10

DQ Treatzza Pizza® and Cake

DQ® Frozen 8" Round Cake, 1 slice (⅛ of cake) 9
DQ® Layered 8" Round Cake, 1 slice (⅛ of cake) 8
Skor® DQ Treatzza Pizza®, 1 serving (1 slice) 4
Smarties® DQ Treatzza Pizza®, 1 serving (1 slice) 4

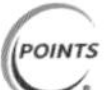

Brazier® Foods Only at Dairy Queen®/Brazier® Stores

DQ® Hamburger, 1 7
DQ® Cheeseburger, 1 8
DQ® Double Cheeseburger, 1 14
DQ® Bacon Double Cheeseburger, 1 ... 17
DQ® Ultiimate Burger, 1 18
Hot Dog, 1 6
Chili 'n Cheese Dog, 1 8
Chicken Breast Fillet Sandwich, 1 9
Grilled Chicken Sandwich, 1 7
Chicken Nuggets, 3 pieces in Kid's Pick Nic!®, 3 pieces 4
Chicken Strip Basket (without gravy and/or dipping sauce), 1 24
French Fries, 1 medium 9
French Fries, 1 large 12
Onion Rings, 1 serving 11

Some Low-*POINT* Ideas

each

½ cup DQ® Chocolate or Vanilla Soft Serve Cone
1 slice Skor® DQ® Treatzza Pizza®
1 slice Smarties® DQ® Treatzza Pizza®

each

1 small Vanilla Cone
1 Dilly Bar®

Only at Dairy Queen®/ Brazier® Stores

3 pieces Kid's Pick Nic!® Chicken Nuggets

1 Hot Dog

each

1 DQ® Hamburger
1 Grilled Chicken Sandwich

D'Angelo Sandwich Shops®

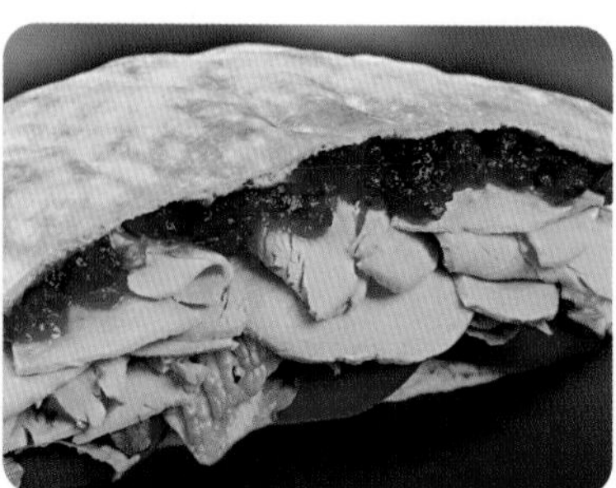

D'Angelo D'Lites® LowFat Sandwiches

	POINTS
Chicken Caesar Salad Honey Wheat Pokket, 1	6
Chicken Caesar Salad Pokket, 1	7
Chicken Caesar Salad Wrap, Regular, 1	8
Chicken Caesar Salad Wrap, Spinach, 1	8
Chicken Caesar Salad Wrap, Tomato, 1	8
Chicken Stir Fry D'Lite Honey Wheat Pokket, 1	7
Chicken Stir Fry D'Lite Pokket, 1	7
Chicken Stir Fry D'Lite Small Sub, 1	8
Chicken Stir Fry D'Lite Wrap, Regular, 1	8
Chicken Stir Fry D'Lite Wrap, Spinach, 1	8
Chicken Stir Fry D'Lite Wrap, Tomato, 1	8
Classic Grilled Veggie Honey Wheat Pokket, 1	5
Classic Grilled Veggie Pokket, 1	6
Classic Grilled Veggie Small Sub, 1	7
Classic Grilled Veggie Wrap, Regular, 1	7
Classic Grilled Veggie Wrap, Spinach, 1	7
Classic Grilled Veggie Wrap, Tomato, 1	7
Fresh Veggie Honey Wheat Pokket, 1	5
Fresh Veggie Pokket, 1	6
Fresh Veggie Small Sub, 1	7
Fresh Veggie Wrap, Regular, 1	6
Fresh Veggie Wrap, Spinach, 1	7
Fresh Veggie Wrap, Tomato, 1	7
Grilled Chicken Filet Honey Wheat Pokket, 1	6
Grilled Chicken Filet Pokket, 1	7
Grilled Chicken Filet Small Sub, 1	8
Grilled Chicken Filet Wrap, Regular, 1	7
Grilled Chicken Filet Wrap, Spinach, 1	8
Grilled Chicken Filet Wrap, Tomato, 1	8
Ham & Cheese Honey Wheat Pokket, 1	5
Ham & Cheese Pokket, 1	6
Ham & Cheese Small Sub, 1	7
Ham & Cheese Wrap, Regular, 1	7
Ham & Cheese Wrap, Spinach, 1	7
Ham & Cheese Wrap, Tomato, 1	7
Roast Beef Honey Wheat Pokket, 1	5
Roast Beef Pokket, 1	6
Roast Beef Small Sub, 1	7
Roast Beef Wrap, Regular, 1	6
Roast Beef Wrap, Spinach, 1	7
Roast Beef Wrap, Tomato, 1	7
Turkey D'Lite Honey Wheat Pokket, 1	5

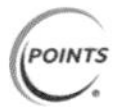

Turkey D'Lite Pokket, 1 6
Turkey D'Lite Small Sub, 1 7
Turkey D'Lite Wrap, Regular, 1 7
Turkey D'Lite Wrap, Spinach, 1 7
Turkey D'Lite Wrap, Tomato, 1 7
Turkey with Cranberry Honey Wheat Pokket, 1 7
Turkey with Cranberry Pokket, 1 8
Turkey with Cranberry Small Sub, 1 9
Turkey with Cranberry Wrap, Regular, 1 9
Turkey with Cranberry Wrap, Spinach, 1 9
Turkey with Cranberry Wrap, Tomato, 1 9

Salads (without Dressing)

Asian Chicken Salad, 1 4
Caesar Salad with Croutons, 1 4
Caesar Salad without Croutons, 1 2
Chicken Caesar Salad with Croutons, 1 6
Chicken Caesar Salad without Croutons, 1 4
Chicken Stir Fry Salad, 1 3
Tossed Salad, 1 0

Salad Dressing

Fat Free Caesar Dressing, 1 packet 0
Lite Buttermilk Ranch Dressing, 2 Tbsp 2

Pita Bread

Honey Wheat Pita Pokket, 1 2
Pita Pokket, 1 1

Meal Ideas

1 Classic Grilled Veggie Honey Wheat Pokket
1 Tossed Salad with 1 packet Fat Free Caesar Dressing

1 Ham & Cheese Honey Wheat Pokket
1 Caesar Salad (without croutons) with 1 packet Fat Free Caesar Dressing

1 regular Roast Beef Wrap
1 Tossed Salad with 2 Tbsp Lite Buttermilk Ranch Dressing

Del Taco®

POINTS

Burgers

Hamburger, 1 6
Cheeseburger, 1 7
Del Cheeseburger™, 1 10
Double Del Cheeseburger™, 1 13
Bacon Double Del Cheeseburger™, 1 15
Bun Taco, 1 10

Burritos

Bean & Cheese Green Burrito, 1 5
Bean & Cheese Red Burrito, 1 5
Chicken Works Burrito, 1 12
Del Beef Burrito™, 1 13
Del Classic Chicken Burrito™, 1 14
Del Combo Burrito, 1 12
Deluxe Combo Burrito™, 1 13
Deluxe Del Beef Burrito™, 1 14
Half Pound Green Burrito, 1 9
Half Pound Red Burrito, 1 9
Macho Beef Burrito™, 1 28
Macho Chicken Burrito™, 1 21
Macho Combo Burrito™, 1 24
Spicy Chicken Burrito, 1 10
Steak Works Burrito, 1 14
Veggie Works Burrito, 1 11

Tacos

Taco, 1 4
Soft Taco, 1 4
Chicken Soft Taco, 1 5
Ultimate Taco, 1 6

POINTS

Big Fat Taco™, 1 7
Big Fat Chicken Taco™, 1 7
Big Fat Steak Taco™, 1 9

Quesadillas

Cheddar Quesadilla, 1 12
Chicken Cheddar Quesadilla, 1 14
Spicy Jack Quesadilla, 1 12
Chicken Spicy Jack Quesadilla, 1 14

Salads

Taco Salad, 1 9
Deluxe Chicken Salad, 1 17
Deluxe Taco Salad™, 1 18

Nachos

Nachos, 1 serving 9
Macho Nachos®, 1 serving 26

Fries

Fries, 1 small serving 5
Fries, 1 regular serving 8
Fries, 1 large serving 12
Macho Fries, 1 serving 17
Chili Cheddar Fries, 1 serving 16
Deluxe Chili Cheddar Fries™, 1 serving 17

Sides

Beans 'n Cheese Cup, 1 serving 5
Rice Cup, 1 serving 3

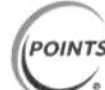

Breakfast

Bacon, 2 slices **1**
Bacon & Egg Quesadilla, 1 .... **11**
Breakfast Burrito, 1 .... **6**
Egg & Cheese Burrito, 1 .... **10**
Macho Bacon & Egg Burrito™, 1 .... **25**
Steak & Egg Burrito, 1 .... **14**

Shakes

Chocolate Shake, 1 small **11**
Chocolate Shake, 1 large **15**
Strawberry Shake, 1 small **9**
Strawberry Shake, 1 large **11**
Vanilla Shake, 1 small **9**
Vanilla Shake, 1 large **12**

MealIdeas

1 Soft Taco
1 serving Beans 'n Cheese Cup

1 Big Fat Taco™
1 serving Rice Cup

1 Hamburger
1 small serving Fries

Denny's®

POINTS

SignatureSkillets® (without choice of bread)

Chicken Fajita Skillet®, 1 serving 20

Meat Lover's Skillet, 1 serving 26

Denny's® FamousSlams

All-American Slam®, without choice of hashed browns, grits, or bread, 1 serving 22

Corned Beef Hash Slam®, 1 serving 18

Farmer's Slam®, without syrup or margarine, 1 serving 30

French Slam®, without syrup or margarine, 1 serving 28

Grand Slam Slugger™, without choice of hashed browns, grits, or bread, 1 serving 23

Lumberjack Slam®, without syrup, margarine, or choice of hashed browns, grits, or bread, 1 serving........25

Original Grand Slam Breakfast®, without syrup or margarine, 1 serving...17

Scram Slam®, without choice of hashed browns, grits, or bread, 1 serving...22

Slim Slam®, without fruit topping, syrup, or margarine (FIT FARE™), 1 serving...9

Omelettes (without choice of hashed browns, grits, or bread)

Ham & Cheddar Omelette with Eggbeaters, 1 serving 12

Ham & Cheddar Omelette, 1 serving ...16

Ultimate Omelette®, 1 serving 16

Veggie-Cheese Omelette, 1 serving 13

POINTS

OtherBreakfastPlatters

Breakfast Dagwood, without choice of bread or potato, 1 serving................36

Country Fried Steak & Eggs, without choice of bread, 1 serving.....11

Moons Over My Hammy®, without choice of potatoes or grits, 1 serving..21

Oatmeal Deluxe (FIT FARE™), 1 serving 9

Sirloin Steak & Eggs, without choice of hashed browns, grits, or bread, 1 serving 17

T-bone Steak & Eggs, without choice of hashed browns, grits, or bread, 1 serving 26

Two Eggs Breakfast, with 4 strips of bacon and hashed browns, without choice of bread, 1 serving.....22

Waffles,Hotcakes&French Toast (without syrup, margarine, bacon, or sausage)

Belgian Waffle, without fruit topping, 1 serving 16

Buttermilk Hotcakes, 1 serving (3 hotcakes) 11

Fabulous French Toast, 1 serving (3) 28

HashedBrowns

Covered & Smothered Hashed Browns, 1 serving 11

Covered Hash Browns, 1 serving 7

Hashed Browns, 1 serving.........................5

POINTS®

Breakfast Sides

Applesauce, 1 serving ... 1
Bacon, 4 strips ... 5
Bagel, dry, 1 ... 5
Banana, 1 serving ... 1
Cantaloupe, 1 serving (¼ melon) ... 0
Country Fried Potatoes, 1 serving ... 9
Cream Cheese, 1 serving ... 3
Dry Cereal (average), 1 serving ... 2
Egg Beaters® Egg Substitute, 1 serving ... 17
Egg, 1 ... 3
English Muffin, 1 ... 2
Fruit Mix, 1 serving ... 1
Grapefruit, ½ ... 0
Grapes, 1 serving ... 1
Grits, 1 serving ... 2
Ham, grilled, 1 slice ... 2
Honeydew, ¼ melon ... 0
Quaker® Oatmeal, 1 serving ... 2
Sausage, 4 links ... 10
Toast, dry, 1 slice ... 2

Syrups & Toppings

Blueberry Topping, 3 oz ... 2
Cherry Topping, 3 oz ... 2
Maple-Flavored Syrup, 3 Tbsp ... 3
Strawberry Topping, 3 oz ... 2
Sugar-Free Maple-Flavored Syrup, 3 Tbsp ... 0
Whipped Cream, 1 dollop ... 1
Whipped Margarine, 1 Tbsp ... 3

POINTS®

Sandwiches (without French fries or condiments that are served on the side)

Albacore Tuna Melt, 1 ... 15
Bacon, Lettuce & Tomato Sandwich, 1 ... 15
BBQ Chicken Sandwich, 1 ... 26
Chicken Ranch Melt, 1 ... 18
Club Sandwich, 1 ... 17
Grilled Chicken Sandwich, 1 ... 10
Ham & Swiss on Rye Sandwich, 1 ... 9
Hoagie Chicken Melt, 1 ... 18
Patty Melt, 1 ... 19
The Super Bird® Sandwich, 1 ... 15
Turkey Breast on Multigrain Bread, 1 ... 5

Burgers (without French fries or condiments that are served on the side)

Bacon-Cheddar Burger, 1 ... 21
BBQ Burger, 1 ... 23
Boca Burger®, 1 ... 13
Buffalo Chicken Sandwich, 1 ... 16
Classic Burger with Cheese, 1 ... 20
Classic Burger, 1 ... 16
Mushroom-Swiss Burger, 1 ... 21

Soups

Chicken Noodle Soup (FIT FARE™), 1 bowl ... 1
Clam Chowder, 1 bowl ... 15
Cream of Broccoli Soup, 1 bowl ... 15
Vegetable Beef Soup (FIT FARE™), 1 bowl ... 1

Denny's®

POINTS

Salads (without bread)

Caesar Side Salad, with dressing, 1 9
Coleslaw, 1 serving 7
Garden Deluxe Salad with Chicken Breast, without dressing (FIT FARE™), 1 5
Garden Deluxe Salad with Fried Chicken Strips, without dressing, 1 10
Garden Salad with Albacore Tuna, with dressing, 1 11
Garden Side Salad, without dressing (FIT FARE™), 1 2
Grilled Chicken Caesar Salad, with dressing, 1 15

Salad Dressings

Blue Cheese Dressing, 1 serving 5
Caesar Dressing, 1 serving 4
Fat Free Ranch Dressing, 1 serving 1
French Dressing, 1 serving 3
Honey Mustard Dressing, 1 serving 4
Low Calorie Italian Dressing (FIT FARE™), 1 serving 0
Ranch Dressing, 1 serving 4
Thousand Island Dressing, 1 serving 3

Appetizers (without dipping sauces or dressings that are served on the side)

Buffalo Chicken Strips, 1 serving (5 strips) 18
Buffalo Wings, 1 serving (12 wings) 21
Chicken Strips, 1 serving (5 strips) 17
Mozzarella Sticks, 1 serving (8 sticks) 17
Sampler™, 1 serving 34
Smothered Cheese Fries, 1 serving 19

POINTS

Dinners (without side dishes or choice of bread)

Chicken Strips, 1 serving 15
Country Fried Steak, 1 serving 7
Fish & Chips, 1 serving 23
Fried Shrimp & Shrimp Scampi, 1 serving 8
Fried Shrimp Dinner, 1 serving (10 shrimp) 5
Grilled Chicken Dinner (FIT FARE™), 1 serving 3
Pot Roast Dinner, with gravy (FIT FARE™), 1 serving 7
Roast Turkey & Stuffing, with gravy (FIT FARE™), 1 serving 8
Shrimp Scampi Skillet Dinner, 1 serving 7
Sirloin Steak Dinner, 1 serving 9
Steak & Shrimp Dinner, 1 serving 16
T-bone Steak Dinner, 1 serving 23

Side Dishes & Herb Toast

Applesauce, 1 serving 1
Baked Potato, plain, with skin, 1 4
Bread Stuffing, plain, 1 serving 2
Carrots in Honey Glaze, 1 serving 1
Corn in Butter Sauce, 1 serving 2
Cottage Cheese, 1 serving 2
French Fries, unsalted, 1 serving 9
Green Beans with Bacon, 1 serving 1
Herb Toast, 2 slices 4
Mashed Potatoes, plain, 1 serving 4
Onion Rings, 1 serving 9
Seasoned Fries, 1 serving 6
Tomato Slices, 3 slices 0

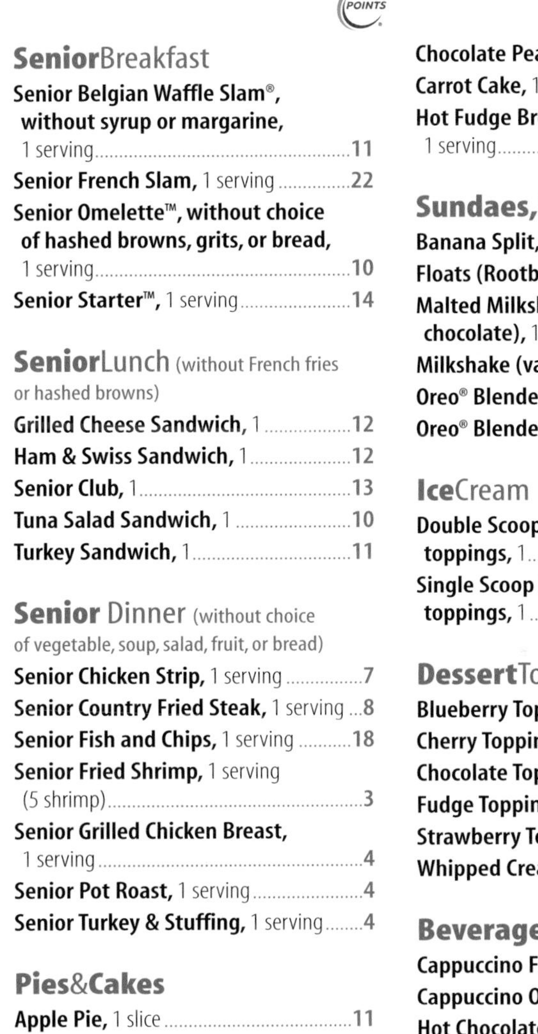

POINTS

Senior Breakfast

Senior Belgian Waffle Slam®, without syrup or margarine, 1 serving ... 11

Senior French Slam, 1 serving ... 22

Senior Omelette™, without choice of hashed browns, grits, or bread, 1 serving ... 10

Senior Starter™, 1 serving ... 14

Senior Lunch (without French fries or hashed browns)

Grilled Cheese Sandwich, 1 ... 12

Ham & Swiss Sandwich, 1 ... 12

Senior Club, 1 ... 13

Tuna Salad Sandwich, 1 ... 10

Turkey Sandwich, 1 ... 11

Senior Dinner (without choice of vegetable, soup, salad, fruit, or bread)

Senior Chicken Strip, 1 serving ... 7

Senior Country Fried Steak, 1 serving ... 8

Senior Fish and Chips, 1 serving ... 18

Senior Fried Shrimp, 1 serving (5 shrimp) ... 3

Senior Grilled Chicken Breast, 1 serving ... 4

Senior Pot Roast, 1 serving ... 4

Senior Turkey & Stuffing, 1 serving ... 4

Pies & Cakes

Apple Pie, 1 slice ... 11

Cheesecake, 1 serving ... 14

POINTS

Chocolate Peanut Butter Pie, 1 slice ... 16

Carrot Cake, 1 slice ... 19

Hot Fudge Brownie a la Mode, 1 serving ... 23

Sundaes, Shakes, & Floats

Banana Split, 1 serving ... 21

Floats (Rootbeer or Cola), 1 ... 6

Malted Milkshake (vanilla/chocolate), 1 ... 14

Milkshake (vanilla/chocolate), 1 ... 13

Oreo® Blender Blaster, 1 ... 21

Oreo® Blender Blaster, 1 kids serving ... 14

Ice Cream

Double Scoop Ice Cream, without toppings, 1 ... 10

Single Scoop Ice Cream, without toppings, 1 ... 5

Dessert Toppings

Blueberry Topping, 1 serving ... 1

Cherry Topping, 1 serving ... 1

Chocolate Topping, 1 serving ... 8

Fudge Topping, 1 serving ... 5

Strawberry Topping, 1 serving ... 1

Whipped Cream, 2 Tbsp ... 1

Beverages

Cappuccino French Vanilla, 1 ... 2

Cappuccino Original Flavor, 1 ... 2

Hot Chocolate, 1 ... 2

Raspberry Iced Tea, 1 ... 2

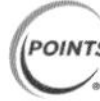

Sauces&Gravies

BBQ Sauce, 1 serving 1
Brown Gravy, 1 serving 0
Chicken Gravy, 1 serving 0
Country Gravy, 1 serving 0
Marinara Sauce, 1 serving 1
Tartar Sauce, 1 serving 6

KidsMeals (without sides)

Burgerlicious™, 1 serving 7
Cheese Burgerlicious™, 1 8
Dennysaur™ Chicken Nuggets, 1 serving 5
Frenchtastic Slam™, 1 serving 12
Jr. Fish and Chips, 1 serving 17
Jr. ShrimpsAhoy!, 1 serving 9
Junior Grand Slam®, 1 serving 10
Pizza Party®, 1 serving 8
Smiley-face Hotcakes with Meat, 1 serving 11
Smiley-face Hotcakes without Meat, 1 serving 7
Star Spangled Hotcakes without Meat, 1 serving 4
The Big Cheese, 1 serving 8

MealIdeas

¼ Cantaloupe
1 serving Quaker® Oatmeal with 3 Tbsp Sugar-Free Maple-Flavored Syrup

1 bowl Chicken Noodle Soup (FIT FARE™)
1 Garden Side Salad (FIT FARE™) with 1 serving Low Calorie Italian Dressing (FIT FARE™)
1 single scoop Ice Cream (without topppings)

1 serving Grilled Chicken Dinner (without bread) (FIT FARE™)
1 serving Plain Mashed Potatoes
1 serving Green Beans with Bacon
1 Raspberry Iced Tea

Dippin' Dots®

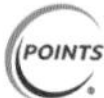

Fat Free Chocolate Ice Cream, 4-oz serving ... 1
Fat Free Chocolate Ice Cream, 5-oz serving ... 1
Fat Free Chocolate Ice Cream, 8-oz serving ... 2
Ice Cream, 4-oz serving ... 4
Ice Cream, 5-oz serving ... 5
Ice Cream, 8-oz serving ... 7
Ice, 4-oz serving ... 1
Ice, 5-oz serving ... 1
Ice, 8-oz serving ... 2
Low Fat Vanilla Ice Cream, 4-oz serving ... 2
Low Fat Vanilla Ice Cream, 5-oz serving ... 3
Low Fat Vanilla Ice Cream, 8-oz serving ... 4
Sherbet, 4-oz serving ... 2
Sherbet, 5-oz serving ... 2
Sherbet, 8-oz serving ... 3
Yogurt, 4-oz serving ... 2
Yogurt, 5-oz serving ... 2
Yogurt, 8-oz serving ... 4

Some Low-*POINT* Ideas

each

4-oz or 5-oz serving Fat Free Chocolate Ice Cream
4-oz or 5-oz serving Ice

each

8-oz serving Fat Free Chocolate Ice Cream
8-oz serving Ice
4-oz or 5-oz serving Sherbet
4-oz or 5-oz serving Yogurt

each

5-oz serving Low Fat Vanilla Ice Cream
8-oz serving Sherbet

Domino's Pizza®

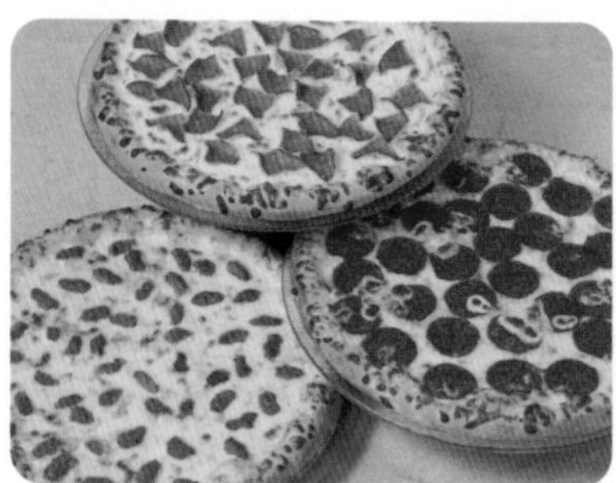

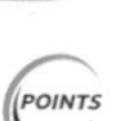

UltimateDeepDishPizza

America's Favorite Pizza Feast™, 1 slice (⅛ of 12" large pizza) 7

America's Favorite Pizza Feast™, 1 slice (⅛ of 14" large pizza) 10

Cheese Pizza, 1 slice (⅛ of 12" medium pizza) 5

Cheese Pizza, 1 slice (⅛ of 14" large pizza) 8

Cheese Pizza, 1 small (6" pizza) 13

Deluxe Pizza Feast™, 1 slice (⅛ of 12" medium pizza) 7

Deluxe Pizza Feast™, 1 slice (⅛ of 14" large pizza) 9

Extra Pepperoni & Extra Cheese Pizza, 1 slice (⅛ of 12" medium pizza) 7

Extra Pepperoni & Extra Cheese Pizza, 1 slice (⅛ of 14" large pizza) 10

ExtravaganZZa Pizza Feast™, 1 slice (⅛ of 12" medium pizza) 7

ExtravaganZZa Pizza Feast™, 1 slice (⅛ of 14" large pizza) 10

Hawaiian Pizza Feast™, 1 slice (⅛ of 12" medium pizza) 6

POINTS

Hawaiian Pizza Feast™, 1 slice (⅛ of 14" large pizza) 9

Meatzza Pizza Feast™, 1 slice (⅛ of 12" medium pizza) 8

Meatzza Pizza Feast™, 1 slice (⅛ of 14" large pizza) 10

Pepperoni Pizza, 1 slice (⅛ of 12" medium pizza) 7

Pepperoni Pizza, 1 slice (⅛ of 14" large pizza) 9

Pepperoni Pizza, 1 small (6" pizza) 17

Vegi Pizza Feast™, 1 slice (⅛ of 12" medium pizza) 6

Vegi Pizza Feast™, 1 slice (⅛ of 14" large pizza) 9

ClassicHandTossedPizza

America's Favorite Pizza Feast™, 1 slice (⅛ of 12" medium pizza) 6

America's Favorite Pizza Feast™, 1 slice (⅛ of 14" large pizza) 8

Cheese Pizza, 1 slice (⅛ of 12" medium pizza) 4

Cheese Pizza, 1 slice (⅛ of 14" large pizza) 5

Deluxe Pizza Feast™, 1 slice (⅛ of 12" medium pizza) 5

Deluxe Pizza Feast™, 1 slice (⅛ of 14" large pizza) 7

Extra Pepperoni & Extra Cheese Pizza, 1 slice (⅛ of 12" medium pizza) 6

Extra Pepperoni & Extra Cheese Pizza, 1 slice (⅛ of 14" large pizza) 8

ExtravaganZZa Pizza Feast™, 1 slice (⅛ of 12" medium pizza) 6

POINTS

ExtravaganZZa Pizza Feast™, 1 slice (⅛ of 14"large pizza) 8

Hawaiian Pizza Feast™, 1 slice (⅛ of 12" medium pizza) 5

Hawaiian Pizza Feast™, 1 slice (⅛ of 14" large pizza) 7

Meatzza Pizza Feast™, 1 slice (⅛ of 12" medium pizza) 6

Meatzza Pizza Feast™, 1 slice (⅛ of 14" large pizza) 9

Pepperoni Pizza, 1 slice (⅛ of 12" medium pizza) 5

Pepperoni Pizza, 1 slice (⅛ of 14" large pizza) 7

Vegi Pizza Feast™, 1 slice (⅛ of 12" medium pizza) 5

Vegi Pizza Feast™, 1 slice (⅛ of 14" large pizza) 6

CrunchyThin**Crust**Pizza

America's Favorite Pizza Feast™, 1 serving (⅛ of 12" medium pizza) 5

America's Favorite Pizza Feast™, 1 serving (⅛ of 14" large pizza) 7

Cheese Pizza, 1 serving (⅛ of 12" medium pizza) 3

Cheese Pizza, 1 serving (⅛ of 14" large pizza) 4

Deluxe Pizza Feast™, 1 serving (⅛ of 12" medium pizza) 4

Deluxe Pizza Feast™, 1 serving (⅛ of 14" large pizza) 6

Extra Pepperoni & Extra Cheese Pizza, 1 serving (⅛ of 12" medium pizza) 5

Extra Pepperoni & Extra Cheese Pizza, 1 serving (⅛ of 14" large pizza) 7

POINTS

ExtravaganZZa Pizza Feast™, 1 serving (⅛ of 12" medium pizza) 5

ExtravaganZZa Pizza Feast™, 1 serving (⅛ of 14" large pizza) 7

Hawaiian Pizza Feast™, 1 serving (⅛ of 12" medium pizza) 4

Hawaiian Pizza Feast™, 1 serving (⅛ of 14" large pizza) 6

Meatzza Pizza Feast™, 1 serving (⅛ of 12" medium pizza) 5

Meatzza Pizza Feast™, 1 serving (⅛ of 14" large pizza) 7

Pepperoni Pizza, 1 serving (⅛ of 12" medium pizza) 4

Pepperoni Pizza, 1 serving (⅛ of 14" large pizza) 6

Vegi Pizza Feast™, 1 serving (⅛ of 12" medium pizza) 4

Vegi Pizza Feast™, 1 serving (⅛ of 14" large pizza) 5

Domino's®Buffalo**Wings**

Barbecue Wings, 1 piece 1

Hot Wings, 1 piece 1

MealIdeas

1 slice of medium Classic Hand Tossed Deluxe Pizza Feast™ Pizza
3 Barbecue Wings

2 servings of medium Crunchy Thin Crust Cheese Pizza
3 Hot Wings

2 slices of medium Classic Hand Tossed Cheese Pizza
3 Barbecue Wings

Eat'nPark®

Appetizers	POINTS
Cheese Fries, 1 serving	21
Cheese Sticks, 1 serving	10
Onion Rings, 1 serving	5
Wings, 1 serving	10
Zucchini, 1 serving	10

Salads/Dressings

Chef Salad, 1 serving	11
Chicken Caesar Salad, 1 serving	5
Chicken Portabella Salad, 1 serving	7
Chicken Salad, 1 serving	10
Fruit Salad with Sherbet, 1 serving	8
Garden Salad, 1 serving	2
House Salad, 1 serving	3
Steak Salad, 1 serving	15
Taco Salad, 1 serving	8
Bleu Cheese Dressing, 1 serving	2
Caesar Dressing, 1 serving	7
French Fat Free Dressing, 1 serving	1
Fruit Salad Dressing, 1 serving	4
Italian Fat Free Dressing, 1 serving	0
Italian Dressing, 1 serving	3
Lite Burgundy Vinaigrette Dressing, 1 serving	1
Thousand Island Dressing, 1 serving	3

Burgers

	POINTS
American Gourmet, 1	19
American Grill, 1	19
Bacon & Cheese, 1	15
Cheese, 1	13
Garden, 1	7
Hamburger, 1	12
Provolone Gourmet, 1	19
Southwest, 1	16
Superburger®, 1	18
Swiss Gourmet, 1	19
Swiss, 1	14
Turkey, 1	11

Breakfast

Bacon, 1 slice	1
Cereal (with milk), 1 serving	7
Cornbeef Hash, 1 serving	8
Egg (fried), 1	3
Eggs (fried), 2	5
Eggs (fried), 3	8
Egg (poached), 1	2
Eggs (poached), 2	4
Eggs (poached with toast & Promise®), 2	8
Egg Beaters® Breakfast, 1 serving	1
Eggs (Benedict), 1 serving	14
French Toast, 1 slice	0
French Toast, 2 slices	1
French Toast, 3 slices	1
Fruit Cup, 1	1
Ham, 1 serving	3
Hash Browns, 1 serving	5
Homefries, 1 serving	5
Oatmeal (plain), 1 serving	2
Oatmeal (with bananas), 1 serving	6
Oatmeal (with fruit), 1 serving	8
Oatmeal (with milk), 1 serving	4
Omelette (bacon & cheese), 1 serving	13
Omelette (cheese), 1 serving	10

POINTS

Omelette (ham & cheese), 1 serving 12
Omelette (supreme), 1 serving 11
Omelette (Western), 1 serving 8
Pancake, 1 4
Pancakes, 2 9
Pancakes, 3 13
Pancake (blueberry), 1 6
Sausage, 1 4
Sausage, 2 7
Sausage, 3 10
Waffles (apple), 1 serving 22
Waffles (Belgian), 1 serving 15

Breads

Bagel (plain), 1 6
Bagel (raisin), 1 6
Bun (hoagie), 1 3
Bun (hot dog), 1 3
Bun (kaiser), 1 4
Bun (superburger), 1 4
Croissant, 1 6
English Muffin, 1 2
Garlic Toast, 1 serving 10
Pita, 1 6
Raisin, 1 serving 1
Rye, 1 serving 1
Sour Dough, 1 serving 1
Toast (buttered), 1 serving 6
Toast (dry), 1 serving 3
Toast (raisin, buttered), 1 serving 6
Toast (rye, buttered), 1 serving 6
Toast (sour dough, buttered), 1 serving 6

POINTS

Toast (whole wheat, buttered), 1 serving 6
White, 1 serving 1
Whole Wheat, 1 serving 1
Yellow, 1 serving 2

Dinners

Chicken & Biscuits, 1 serving 12
Chicken Breast (stuffed), 1 serving 9
Chicken Fillets, 5 13
Chicken Milano, 1 serving 5
Chicken Naturelle, 1 serving 3
Chicken Parmesan (marinara), 1 serving 19
Chicken Parmesan (meat), 1 serving 20
Chicken Stir-Fry, 1 serving 12
Chicken, 3 pieces 29
Cod (breaded), 1 serving 22
Country Fried Chicken Steak, 1 serving 19
Fish & Chips, 1 serving 25
Ground Sirloin, 1 serving 11
Ham Steak, 1 serving 4
Island Cod, 1 serving 4
Liver, 1 serving 6
Nantucket Cod, 1 serving 7
Salisbury Steak, 1 serving 11
Salmon, 1 serving 5
Scallops, 1 serving 10
Scrod (baked), 1 serving 11
Scrod (Floridian), 1 serving 2
Scrod (Maryland), 1 serving 11
Spaghetti Marinara, 1 serving 12
Spaghetti Meat Sauce, 1 serving 17

POINTS

Dinners (con't)

Top Sirloin, 1 serving 8
Turkey, 1 serving 8
Veal Parmesan Marinara, 1 serving 12
Veal Parmesan Meat Sauce, 1 serving 18
Whitefish (breaded), 1 serving 18
Ziti with Meatballs (marinara), 1 serving 18
Ziti with Meatballs (meat), 1 serving 22

Sandwiches

Bacon Turkey Swiss, 1 13
BLT, 1 7
Chicken (breaded), 1 12
Chicken (spicy), 1 7
Chicken Bacon Deluxe, 1 13
Chicken Fiesta, 1 7
Chicken, 1 7
Cod (breaded), 1 15
Croissant (chicken salad), 1 15
Croissant (tuna), 1 14
Croissant (turkey), 1 9
Dutch Ham & Swiss, 1 13
Grilled Cheese, 1 13
Hot Roast Beef, 1 6
Pita (chicken fajita), 1 13
Pita (tuna), 1 14
Pita (turkey), 1 9
Reuben, 1 18
Shredded Pot Roast, 1 13
Steak'n Cheese, 1 19
Tuna Melt, 1 15
Turkey Club, 1 19

POINTS

Turkey Pastrami, 1 17
Whitefish (breaded), 1 18

Seniors

Chicken Fillet, 4 pieces 10
Chicken, 2 pieces 24
Cod (breaded), 1 serving 11
Fish (breaded), 1 serving 11
French Toast, 1 serving 9
Roast Beef, 1 serving 6
Scrod (baked), 1 serving 9
Scrod (Floridian), 1 serving 2
Spaghetti (marinara), 1 serving 6
Spaghetti (meat), 1 serving 8
Turkey (hot), 1 serving 5

Sides

Applesauce, 1 serving 2
Banana, 1 medium 2
Banana, 1 large 2
Bean Soup, 1 cup 2
Bean Soup, 1 bowl 6
Beef Noodle Soup, 1 cup 2
Beef Noodle Soup, 1 bowl 5
Broccoli Soup, 1 cup 5
Broccoli Soup, 1 bowl 9
Buttered Noodles, 1 serving 6
Cheese Soup, 1 cup 5
Cheese Soup, 1 bowl 10
Chicken Noodle Soup, 1 cup 3
Chicken Noodle Soup, 1 bowl 6
Chicken Rice Soup, 1 cup 2
Chicken Rice Soup, 1 bowl 3
Chili, 1 cup 2

	POINTS
Chili, 1 bowl	4
Clam Chowder, 1 cup	4
Clam Chowder, 1 bowl	7
Coleslaw, 1 serving	5
Cottage Cheese, 1 serving	2
French Fries, 1 serving	8
Fresh Strawberries, 1 cup	0
Gravy (beef), 1 serving	0
Gravy (turkey), 1 serving	1
Kielbasa Soup, 1 cup	1
Kielbasa Soup, 1 bowl	3
Macaroni & Cheese, 1 serving	3
Minestroni Soup, 1 cup	1
Minestroni Soup, 1 bowl	3
Mushroom Barley Soup, 1 cup	1
Mushroom Barley Soup, 1 bowl	2
Nacho Chips, 1 serving	3
Onion Rings, 10	3
Potato (baked), 1	3
Potato (scalloped), 1 serving	5
Potato (whipped), 1 serving	7
Potato Soup, 1 cup	5
Potato Soup, 1 bowl	8
Rice (Mexican), 1 serving	2
Rice (white), 1 serving	3
Rice Pilaf, 1 serving	3
Rice Pudding, 1 serving	3
Stuffed Pepper Soup, 1 cup	2
Stuffed Pepper Soup, 1 bowl	5
Sugar Snap Peas, 1 serving	0
Vegetable Beef Barley, 1 cup	2
Vegetable Beef Barley, 1 bowl	4
Vegetables (mixed), 1 serving	0
Vegetarian Pasta, 1 cup	1
Vegetarian Pasta, 1 bowl	2
Vegetarian Soup, 1 cup	1
Vegetarian Soup, 1 bowl	3
Wedding Soup, 1 cup	2
Wedding Soup, 1 bowl	4

Bakery

	POINTS
Bear Claw, 1	12
Biscuit, 1	1
Biscuit (cheese), 1	3
Boston Brown Bread, 2 slices	6
Cinnamon Biscuit, 1 (mini)	3
Cinnamon Bun, 1	6
Cookie (chocolate chip), 1	5
Cookie (Christmas), 1	6
Cookie (Easter), 1	6
Cookie (Halloween), 1	8
Cookie (macadamia nut), 1	6
Cookie (shamrock), 1	7
Cookie (Smiley®), 1	7
Cookie (steeler/penguin/pirate), 1	7
Cookie (valentine), 1	6
Cornbread, 1 serving	2
Crumby Buns, 1	5
Honey Bun, 1	4
Muffin (apple raisin), 1	5
Muffin (banana nut), 1	6
Muffin (blueberry), 1	5
Muffin (chocolate nut), 1	7
Muffin (corn), 1	5
Muffin (cranberry), 1	6
Muffin (oatbran apple raisin), 1	6
Muffin (oatbran), 1	7
Muffin (pumpkin raisin), 1	6

POINTS

Bakery (con't)

Muffin (strawberry creme), 1 6
Muffin (strawberry filled), 1 6
SnoTop, 1 2
Sticky Loaf, 1 7

Desserts

Banana Fudge Sensation, 1 serving 22
Caramel Nut Fudge Sensation, 1 serving 25
Cheesecake, 1 slice 13
Cheesecake (with strawberries), 1 slice 18
Cookie Fudge Fantasy, 1 serving 28
Grilled Sticky Ala Mode, 1 serving 17
Grilled Sticky Loaf, 1 serving 12
Ice Cream, 2 scoops 7
Pie (apple), 1 slice 11
Pie (apple cranberry), 1 slice 16
Pie (apple reduced fat), 1 slice 7
Pie (banana), 1 slice 10
Pie (blackberry), 1 slice 11
Pie (blueberry), 1 slice 10
Pie (cherry), 1 slice 11
Pie (chocolate peanut butter), 1 slice 14
Pie (coconut cream), 1 slice 12
Pie (lemon meringue), 1 slice 6
Pie (oreo cream), 1 slice 12
Pie (peach lite), 1 slice 6
Pie (peachberry), 1 slice 9
Pie (pecan), 1 slice 16
Pie (pumpkin), 1 slice 9
Pie (shell, baked), 1 serving 5
Pie (strawberry), 1 slice 8

POINTS

Pudding (sugar free chocolate), 1 serving 2
Sherbet (plain), 1 serving 2
Strawberry fudge delight, 1 serving 26
Strawberry shortcake, 1 serving 16
Sundae (apple), 1 junior 7
Sundae (apple), 1 serving 13
Sundae (chocolate), 1 junior 6
Sundae (chocolate), 1 serving 12
Sundae (hot fudge), 1 junior 8
Sundae (hot fudge), 1 serving 15
Sundae (strawberry), 1 serving 14
Sundae (tinroof), 1 serving 19
Yogurt, 1 serving 1

MealIdeas

1 serving Ham Steak or Island Cod
1 serving Mixed Vegetables
1 serving Sugar Free Chocolate Pudding

1 serving Chicken Naturelle
1 serving Garden Salad with
 1 serving French Fat Free Dressing
1 serving Cornbread

1 serving Chicken Caesar Salad with
 1 serving Italian Fat Free Dressing
1 Kaiser Bun

El Pollo Loco

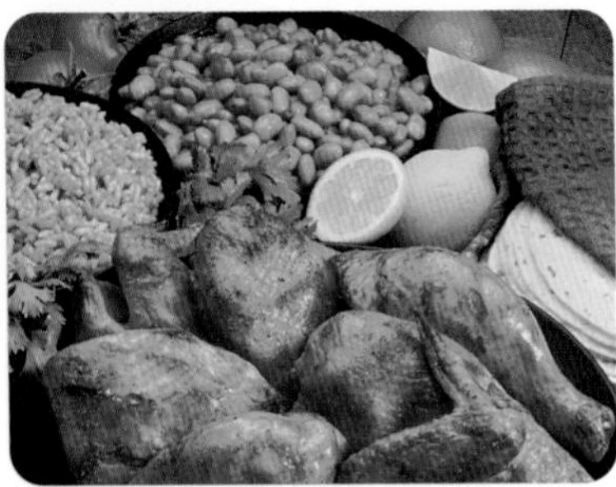

POINTS®

Flame-Broiled Chicken

Breast, 1 serving 4
Leg, 1 serving 2
Thigh, 1 serving 5
Wing, 1 serving 3

Specialty

Chicken Tostada Salad (without Shell & Sour Cream), 1 6

Bowl

Pollo Bowl®, 1 10

Burritos

BRC, 1 11
Classic Chicken™, 1 13

Tacos

Chicken Soft Taco, 1 6
Taco al Carbon, 1 4

POINTS®

Tortillas

6" Corn Tortilla, 1 1
6½" Flour Tortilla, 1 3

Side Dishes (individual)

Cole Slaw, 1 serving 5
Corn Cobbette, 1 1
Fresh Vegetables, 1 serving 1
Garden Salad, 1 2
Mashed Potatoes, 1 serving 2
Pinto Beans, 1 serving 3
Spanish Rice, 1 serving 3

Dressings

Light Italian, 1 serving 0

Condiments

Avocado Salsa, 1 serving 0
House Salsa, 1 serving 0
Jalapeño Hot Sauce, 1 packet 0
Pico de Gallo Salsa, 1 serving 0
Spicy Chipotle Salsa, 1 serving 0

MealIdeas

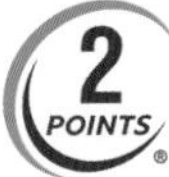

2 6" Corn Tortillas
1 serving Avocado Salsa
1 serving Pico de Gallo Salsa

1 Taco al Carbon
1 Garden Salad with
1 serving Light Italian Dressing

1 serving Flame-Broiled Chicken Breast
1 serving Mashed Potaotes
1 serving of Fresh Vegetables

El Torito®

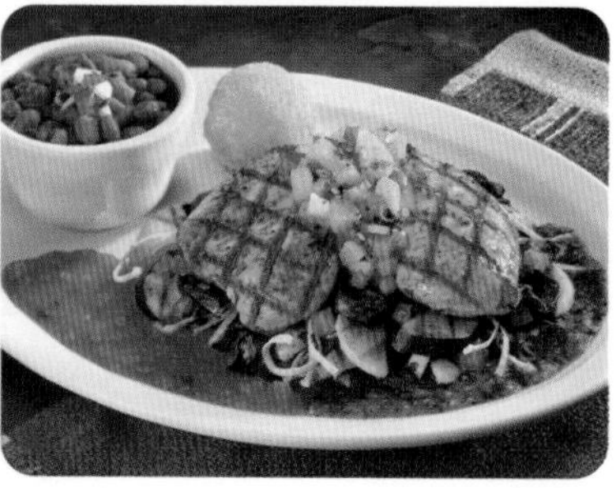

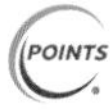

Entrées

Grilled Chicken Breast Fajitas (without Rice, Sonora Beans, Sweet Corn Cake and tortillas), 1 serving....19

Grilled Chicken Caesar Salad (without dressing), 1 serving....11

(If Shrimp is substituted for Chicken), 1 serving....12

Grilled Chicken Quesadilla Lite, 1 serving....13

Pollo Fresco (without Frijoles de la Olla and Sweet Corn Cake), 1 serving....15

Sonora Burrito Lite, 1 serving....18

Spinach Enchiladas (without Rice, Sonora Beans and Sweet Corn Cake), 1 serving....11

Tostada Grande - Chicken (without Guacamole, Sour Cream and tostada), 1 serving....12

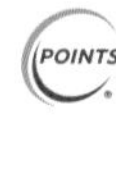

Salad Dressing & Sides

Cilantro-Pepita Dressing™, 1 serving....9

Frijoles de la Olla, 1 serving....2

Guacamole, 1 serving....1

Rice, 1 serving....3

Sonora Beans, 1 serving....3

Sour Cream, 1 serving....2

Sweet Corn Cake, 1 serving....2

Meal Ideas

1 serving Grilled Chicken Caesar Salad (without dressing)

1 serving Grilled Shrimp Caesar Salad (without dressing)

1 serving Tostada Grande – Chicken (without Sour Cream and tostada)
1 serving Guacamole

Fazoli's® Restaurants

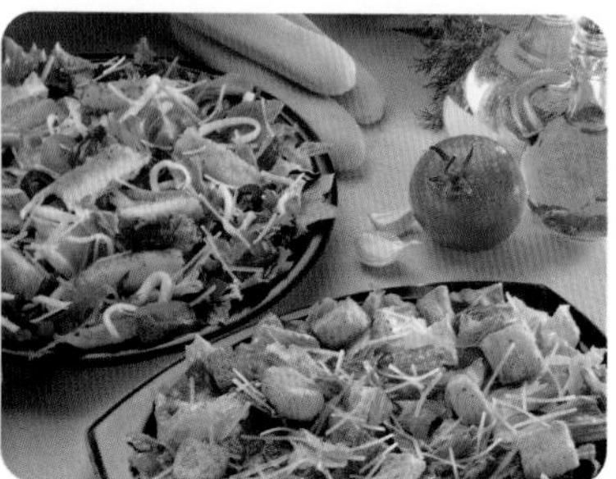

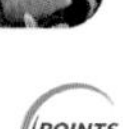

Pasta

Baked Spaghetti Parmesan, 1 serving 15
Baked Ziti, 1 small serving 10
Broccoli Fettuccine Alfredo, 1 small serving 12
Broccoli Lasagna, 1 serving 9
Cheese Ravioli with Meat Sauce, 1 serving 11
Cheese Ravioli with Tomato Sauce, 1 serving 10
Fettuccine Alfredo, 1 small serving 11
Lasagna, 1 serving 10
Sampler Platter, 1 serving 15
Spaghetti with Meat Sauce, 1 small serving 9
Spaghetti with Meat Sauce, 1 regular serving 14
Spaghetti with Tomato Sauce, 1 small serving 8
Spaghetti with Tomato Sauce, 1 regular serving 12

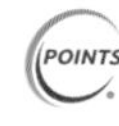

Pizza

Cheese Pizza, 1 serving 10
Pepperoni Pizza, 1 serving 12

PaniniSandwiches

Chicken Pesto Panini Sandwich, 1 11
Ham & Swiss Panini Sandwich, 1 14
Italian Deli Panini Sandwich, 1 15
Parmesan Ranch Chicken Panini Sandwich, 1 15

Soup

Minestrone Soup, 1 serving 2

Salads

Caesar Side Salad, 1 serving 5
Chicken & Pasta Caesar Salad, 1 serving 11
Chicken Caesar Salad, 1 serving 10
Chicken Finger Salad with Bacon Honey Mustard Dressing, 1 serving 10
Chicken Finger Salad, 1 serving 4
Garden Salad with Balsamic Vinaigrette Dressing, 1 serving 3
Garden Salad, 1 serving 0
Pasta Salad, 1 serving 13

Breadsticks

Breadstick - Dry, 1 serving 2
Breadstick, 1 serving 3

Desserts

Cheesecake, Chocolate Chip, 1 serving 8
Cheesecake, Plain, 1 serving 8
Lemon Ice, 1 serving 4
Strawberry Topping, 1 serving 1

MealIdeas

1 serving Minestrone Soup
1 serving Garden Salad with Balsamic Vinaigrette Dressing
1 serving Dry Breadstick

1 small serving Spaghetti with Tomato Sauce
1 serving Garden Salad with Balsamic Vinaigrette Dressing

1 serving Broccoli Lasagna
1 serving Garden Salad
1 serving Breadstick

Freshëns® Frozen Treats

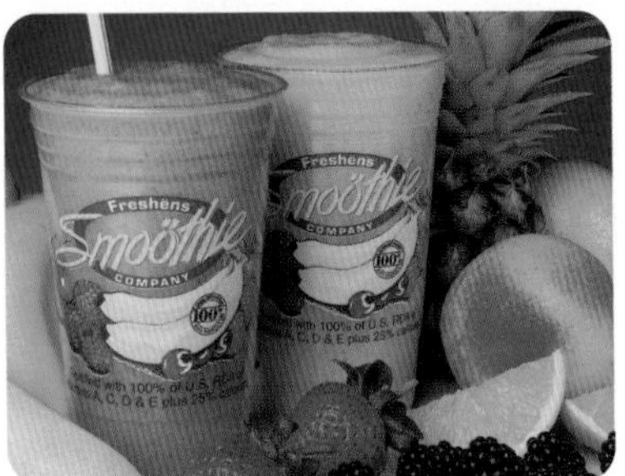

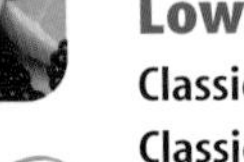

YogurtSmoöthies

Blueberry Sunset, 1 serving 7
Jamaican Jammer, 1 serving 9
Peachy Pineapple, 1 serving 8
Pina Collider, 1 serving 11
Raspberry Rapture, 1 serving 10
Raspberry Rocker, 1 serving 9
Strawberry Squeeze, 1 serving 7

FruitJuice**Smoöthies**

Blueberry Wave, 1 serving 6
Caribbean Craze, 1 serving 6
Peach Sunset, 1 serving 7
Pineapple Passion, 1 serving 8
Raspberry Rhapsody, 1 serving 6
Raspberry Rhumba, 1 serving 7
Strawberry Shooter, 1 serving 5

OrangeSmoöthies

Aruba Orange, 1 serving 8
Orange Shooter, 1 serving 7
Orange Sunrise, 1 serving 8
Orange Wave, 1 serving 8

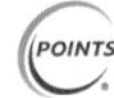

CoffeeSmoöthies

Caramel Coffee, 1 serving 9
Mocha Coffee, 1 serving 8
Oreo® Coffee, 1 serving 11
Original Coffee, 1 serving 7

LowfatFrozen**Yogurt**

Classic Chocolate, 5 fl oz 3
Classic Vanilla, 5 fl oz 3
White Chocolate Mousse, 5 fl oz 3

NonfatFrozen**Yogurt**

Butter Pecan, 5 fl oz 2
Coffee, 5 fl oz 3
Dutch Chocolate, 5 fl oz 3
Flan De Leche, 5 fl oz 3
Georgia Peach, 5 fl oz 3
Key Lime, 5 fl oz 3
New York Cheesecake, 5 fl oz 3
Strawberry, 5 fl oz 2
Vanilla, 5 fl oz 3

Nonfat/No**Sugar** Frozen **Yogurt**

Praline Pecan, 5 fl oz 3
Raspberry Royale, 5 fl oz 2
Strawberries-N-Cream, 5 fl oz 2
Vanilla Fudge, 5 fl oz 2

Some Low-*POINT* Ideas

each

5 fl oz Nonfat Butter Pecan or Strawberry Frozen Yogurt
5 fl oz Nonfat/No Sugar Raspberry Royale, Strawberries-N-Cream, or Vanilla Fudge Frozen Yogurt

each

5 fl oz Lowfat Classic Chocolate or Vanilla Frozen Yogurt
5 fl oz Lowfat White Chocolate Mousse Frozen Yogurt
5 fl oz Nonfat Coffee, Dutch Chocolate, Flan De Leche, Georgia Peach, Key Lime, New York Cheesecake, or Vanilla Frozen Yogurt
5 fl oz Nonfat/No Sugar Praline Pecan Frozen Yogurt

1 serving Strawberry Shooter Fruit Juice Smoöthie

Godfather's Pizza®

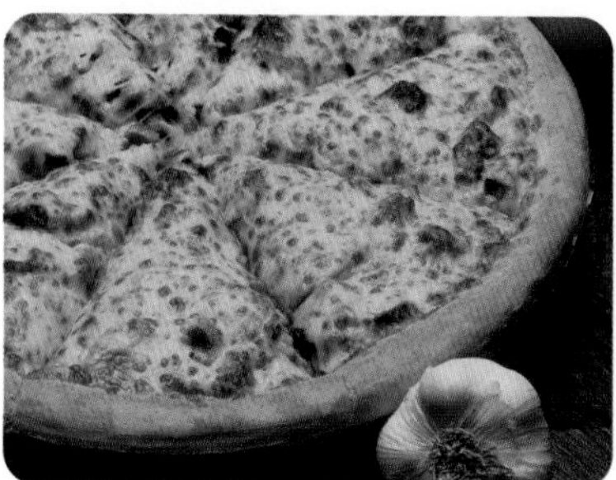

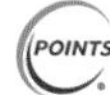

OriginalCrustPizza

Cheese Pizza, 1 slice (⅛ of medium pizza) 5

Cheese Pizza, 1 slice (1⁄10 of large pizza) 6

Combo Pizza, 1 slice (⅛ of medium pizza) 7

Combo Pizza, 1 slice (1⁄10 of large pizza) 8

Veggie Pizza, 1 slice (⅛ of medium pizza) 5

Veggie Pizza, 1 slice (1⁄10 of large pizza) 6

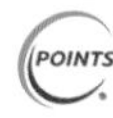

GoldenCrustPizza

Cheese Pizza, 1 slice (⅛ of medium pizza) 5

Cheese Pizza, 1 slice (1⁄10 of large pizza) 5

Combo Pizza, 1 slice (⅛ of medium pizza) 6

Combo Pizza, 1 slice (1⁄10 of large pizza) 6

Veggie Pizza, 1 slice (⅛ of medium pizza) 5

Veggie Pizza, 1 slice (1⁄10 of large pizza) 5

Some Low-*POINT* Ideas

each

1 slice of medium Original Crust Cheese Pizza
1 slice of medium Original Crust Veggie Pizza
1 slice of medium or large Golden Crust Cheese Pizza
1 slice of medium or large Golden Crust Veggie Pizza

each

1 slice of large Original Crust Cheese Pizza
1 slice of large Original Crust Veggie Pizza
1 slice of medium or large Golden Crust Combo Pizza

1 slice of medium Original Crust Combo Pizza

Häagen-Dazs® Shops

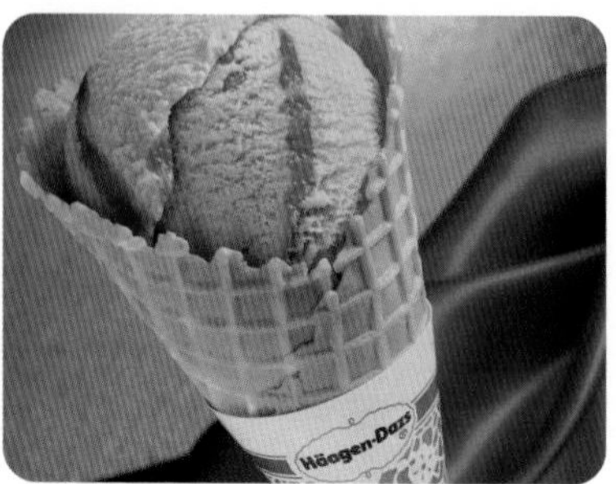

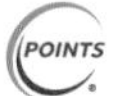

IceCream

Baileys® Irish Cream Ice Cream, ½ cup....7
Belgian Chocolate Chocolate Ice Cream, ½ cup....8
Brownies a la Mode Ice Cream, ½ cup....7
Butter Pecan Ice Cream, ½ cup....8
Cappuccino Commotion® Ice Cream, ½ cup....8
Chocolate Chocolate Chip Ice Cream, ½ cup....7
Chocolate Ice Cream, ½ cup....6
Chocolate Swiss Almond Ice Cream, ½ cup....7
Coffee Ice Cream, ½ cup....6
Coffee Mocha Chip Ice Cream, ½ cup....7
Cookie Dough Dynamo® Ice Cream, ½ cup....8
Cookies & Cream Ice Cream, ½ cup....7
Deep Chocolate Peanut Butter Ice Cream, ½ cup....8
Dulce De Leche Caramel Ice Cream, ½ cup....7

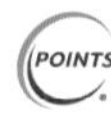

Macadamia Brittle Ice Cream, ½ cup....7
Mint Chip Ice Cream, ½ cup....7
Pralines & Cream Ice Cream, ½ cup....7
Rum Raisin Ice Cream, ½ cup....7
Strawberry Ice Cream, ½ cup....6
Vanilla Chocolate Chip Ice Cream, ½ cup....7
Vanilla Ice Cream, ½ cup....6
Vanilla Swiss Almond Ice Cream, ½ cup....7

CoatedIce**Cream**Bars

Vanilla & Almonds Ice Cream Bar, 1....10
Vanilla & Milk Chocolate Ice Cream Bar, 1....9

UncoatedIce**Cream**Bar

Vanilla Ice Cream Bar, 1....5

Sorbet (hard scoop)

Mango Sorbet, ½ cup....2
Orange Sorbet, ½ cup....2
Raspberry Sorbet, ½ cup....2

Some Low-*POINT* Ideas

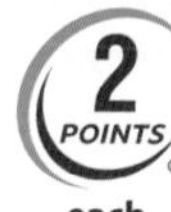

each

½ cup Mango Hard Scoop Sorbet
½ cup Orange Hard Scoop Sorbet
½ cup Raspberry Hard Scoop Sorbet

1 Uncoated Vanilla Ice Cream Bar

each

½ cup Chocolate Ice Cream
½ cup Coffee Ice Cream
½ cup Strawberry Ice Cream
½ cup Vanilla Ice Cream

Hardee's®

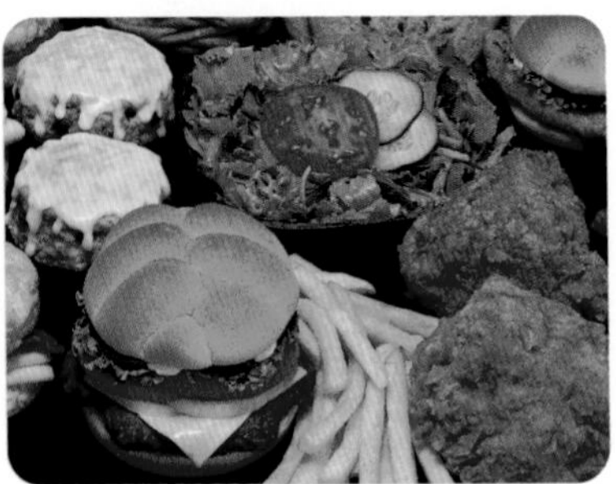

POINTS

Hamburgers&Sandwiches

Hamburger, 1 small 6
Cheeseburger, 1 small 8
Double Cheeseburger, 1 12
All Star, 1 17
Famous Star™ Burger, 1 14
Famous Star™ Burger, with cheese, 1 17
Frisco™ Burger, 1 19
Monster Burger®, 1 26
Mushroom 'N' Swiss™ Burger, 1 12
⅓ Lb. Bacon Thickburger, 1 21
⅓ Lb. Cheeseburger, 1 15
⅓ Lb. Chili Cheese Thickburger, 1 22
⅓ Lb. Thickburger, 1 19
½ Lb. Grilled Sourdough, 1 26
½ Lb. Six Dollar, 1 23
⅔ Lb. Bacon Thickburger, 1 30
⅔ Lb. Thickburger, 1 28
Big Chicken Fillet Sandwich, 1 17
Big Roast Beef™ Sandwich, 1 10
Chicken Fillet Sandwich, 1 10

POINTS

Fisherman's Fillet™ Sandwich, 1 13
Grilled Chicken Sandwich, 1 8
Hot Dog (with condiments), 1 12
Hot Ham 'N' Cheese™ Sandwich, 1 7
Monster Roast Beef, 1 15
Regular Roast Beef Sandwich, 1 8
Slammer with Cheese, 1 8
Slammer, 1 7
Super Star® Burger, 1 20
Super Star® Burger, with cheese, 1 23
The Six Dollar Burger™, 1 23

FriedChicken

Chicken Strips, 3 pieces 3
Chicken Strips, 5 pieces 5
Fried Chicken Breast, 1 (as served with skin) 9
Fried Chicken Leg, 1 (as served with skin) 4
Fried Chicken Thigh, 1 (as served with skin) 8
Fried Chicken Wing, 1 (as served with skin) 5

SideOrders

Coleslaw, 1 small serving 6
Crispy Curls™ Potatoes, 1 regular serving 8
Crispy Curls™ Potatoes, 1 large serving 13
Crispy Curls™ Potatoes, 1 jumbo serving 14
French Fries, 1 regular serving 8
French Fries, 1 large serving 11

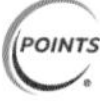

French Fries, 1 jumbo serving 12
Gravy, 1 small serving (3 Tbsp) 0
Mashed Potatoes, without gravy, 1 small serving 1

Breakfast

Apple Cinnamon 'N' Raisin™ Biscuit, 1 6
Bacon, Egg & Cheese Biscuit, 1 13
Biscuit 'N' Gravy™, 1 serving 13
Chicken Biscuit, 1 14
Cinnamon 'N Raisin™ Biscuit, 1 9
Country Ham Biscuit, 1 11
Frisco™ Breakfast Sandwich (Ham), 1 11
Ham Biscuit, 1 10
Jelly Biscuit, 1 11
Made From Scratch™ Biscuit, 1 10
Omelet Biscuit, 1 14
Pork Chop Biscuit, 1 12
Regular Hash Rounds™, 1 serving (16 pieces) 6
Sausage & Egg Biscuit, 1 16
Sausage Biscuit, 1 14
Steak Biscuit, 1 14
Sunrise Croissant (Bacon), 1 10
Sunrise Croissant (Ham), 1 10
Sunrise Croissant (Sausage), 1 15

Desserts

Apple Turnover, 1 6
Chocolate Chip Cookie, 1 9
Peach Cobbler, 1 small serving 7

MealIdeas

1 Hot Ham 'N' Cheese™ Sandwich
1 small serving Mashed Potatoes with 1 small serving Gravy

1 Regular Roast Beef Sandwich
1 small serving Mashed Potatoes with 1 small serving Gravy

1 Fried Chicken Leg (with skin)
1 small serving Coleslaw
1 small serving Mashed Potatoes with 1 small serving Gravy

JACK IN THE BOX®

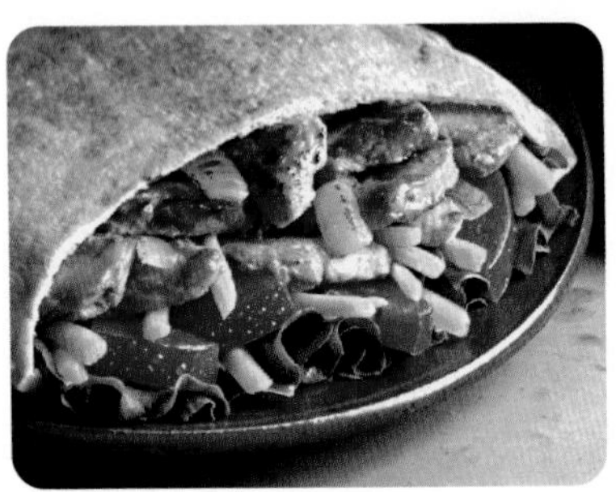

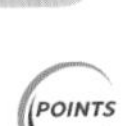

Burgers

Hamburger, 1 small 7
Hamburger with Cheese, 1 small 9
SOURDOUGH JACK®, 1 17
JUMBO JACK®, 1 14
JUMBO JACK® with Cheese, 1 16
Jack's Western Cheeseburger, 1 16
Chili Cheeseburger, 1 10
Double Cheeseburger, 1 14
Big Cheeseburger, 1 17
Ultimate Cheeseburger, 1 25
Junior Bacon Cheeseburger, 1 14
Bacon Bacon Cheeseburger, 1 23
Bacon Ultimate Cheeseburger, 1 28

Sandwiches

Chicken Fajita Pita, 1 7
Chicken Sandwich, 1 10
Chicken Supreme, 1 20
Chipotle Chicken, 1 9
Grilled Chicken Fillet, 1 10
JACK'S SPICY CHICKEN®, 1 15

POINTS

Philly Cheesesteak, 1 12
Sourdough Grilled Chicken Club, 1 12

Tacos

Taco, 1 4
Monster Taco, 1 6

Teriyaki Bowl

Chicken Teriyaki Bowl, 1 11

Salads & Salad Dressings

Side Salad, without dressing, 1 1
Bleu Cheese Dressing, 1 packet (approximately 4 Tbsp) 7
Buttermilk House Dressing, 1 packet (approximately 4 Tbsp) 9
Low-Calorie Italian Dressing, 1 packet (approximately 4 Tbsp) 0
Thousand Island Dressing, 1 packet (approximately 4 Tbsp) 4
Croutons, 1 serving 1

Side Orders

French Fries, 1 small 7
French Fries, 1 medium 9
French Fries, Super Scoop, 1 large 13
Seasoned Curly Fries, 1 serving 9
Chili Cheese Curly Fries, 1 serving 15
Onion Rings, 1 serving 12

Breakfast

BREAKFAST JACK®, 1 7
EXTREME SAUSAGE® Sandwich, 1 18
French Toast Sticks, without syrup, 1 serving 10

POINTS

Syrup, 1 packet (3 Tbsp) 3
Hash Browns, 1 serving 3
Sausage Biscuit, 1 9
Sausage Croissant, 1 17
Sausage, Egg & Cheese Biscuit, 1 20
Sourdough Breakfast Sandwich, 1 11
Supreme Croissant, 1 14
Ultimate Breakfast Sandwich, 1 18

FingerFoods

Bacon Cheddar Potato Wedges, 1 serving 20
Chicken Breast Pieces, 5 pieces 8
Cheese Sticks, 3 6
Cheese Sticks, 5 9
Egg Roll, 1 3
Egg Rolls, 3 9
Fish & Chips, 1 serving 14
Stuffed Jalapeños, 3 pieces 5
Stuffed Jalapeños, 7 pieces 12
Taquitos, 3 7
Taquitos, 5 11
Barbecue Dipping Sauce, 1 packet (2 Tbsp) 1
Buttermilk House Dipping Sauce, 1 packet (2 Tbsp) 4
Frank's Red Hot® Buffalo Dipping Sauce, 1 packet (2 Tbsp) 0
Marinara Sauce, 1 serving 0
Salsa, 1 serving 0
Sour Cream, 1 serving 2
Soy Sauce, 1 serving 0
Sweet & Sour Dipping Sauce, 1 packet (2 Tbsp) 1

POINTS

Shakes

Cappuccino Ice Cream Shake, 1 regular 15
Chocolate Ice Cream Shake, 1 regular 15
Oreo® Cookie Ice Cream Shake, 1 regular 16
Strawberry Banana Ice Cream Shake, 1 serving 16
Strawberry Ice Cream Shake, 1 regular 15
Vanilla Ice Cream Shake, 1 regular 14

Desserts

Apple Turnover, 1 7
Cheesecake, 1 serving 8
Double Fudge Cake, 1 serving 6

Meal Ideas

1 Taco
1 Side Salad with
1 packet Low-Calorie Italian Dressing

1 small Hamburger
1 Side Salad with
1 packet Low-Calorie Italian Dressing

1 Breakfast Jack®
1 serving Hash Browns

Jamba Juice®

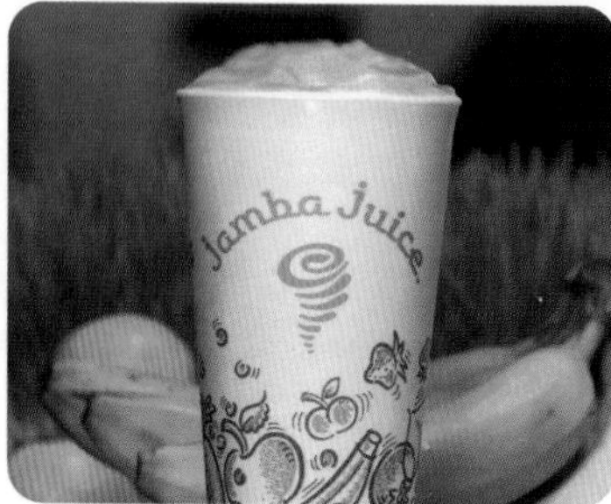

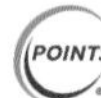

Smoothie

	POINTS
Banana Berry™, 16 fl oz	5
Caribbean Passion®, 16 fl oz	5
Cranberry Craze®, 16 fl oz	5
Kiwi Berry Burner®, 16 fl oz	5
Mango-A-Go-Go™, 16 fl oz	6
Orange Dream Machine™, 16 fl oz	8
Orange Mango Zoom™, 16 fl oz	5
Orange-A-Peel™, 16 fl oz	5
PowerBoost®, 16 fl oz	5
Strawberries Wild™, 16 fl oz	5

JuiceBoost™

	POINTS
Fiber Juice Boost™, 1 Tbsp	0
Protein Juice Boost™, 1 small scoop	1

Some Low-*POINT* Ideas

5 POINTS® each

1 Banana Berry™ Smoothie
1 Caribbean Passion® Smoothie
1 Cranberry Craze® Smoothie
1 Kiwi Berry Burner® Smoothie
1 Orange Mango Zoom™ Smoothie
1 Orange-A-Peel™ Smoothie
1 PowerBoost® Smoothie
1 Strawberries Wild® Smoothie

6 POINTS®

1 Mango-A-Go-Go™ Smoothie

8 POINTS®

1 Orange Dream Machine™ Smoothie

Jersey Mike's® Subs

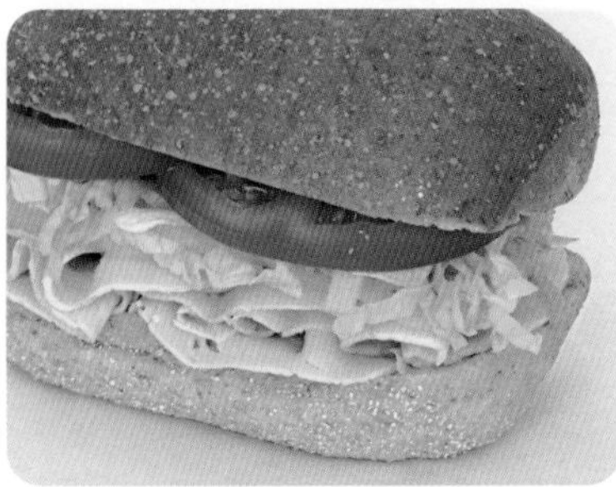

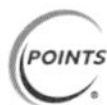

MiniMike**Cold**Subs (all subs include onions, lettuce, and tomato)

Ham on Wheat, one 4-inch 5
Ham on White, one 4-inch 5
Ham and Turkey on Wheat, one 4-inch 5
Ham and Turkey on White, one 4-inch 5
Roast Beef on Wheat, one 4-inch 6
Roast Beef on White, one 4-inch 6
Turkey on Wheat, one 4-inch 4
Turkey on White, one 4-inch 5
Veggie on Wheat, one 4-inch 3
Veggie on White, one 4-inch 3

Note: Available at participating locations.

Some Low-*POINT* Ideas

each

One 4-inch Mini Mike Veggie on Wheat Cold Sub
One 4-inch Mini Mike Veggie on White Cold Sub

One 4-inch Mini Mike Turkey on Wheat Cold Sub

each

One 4-inch Mini Mike Ham on Wheat Cold Sub
One 4-inch Mini Mike Ham on White Cold Sub
One 4-inch Mini Mike Ham and Turkey on Wheat Cold Sub
One 4-inch Mini Mike Ham and Turkey on White Cold Sub
One 4-inch Mini Mike Turkey on White Cold Sub

Jreck Subs®

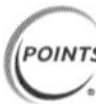

LowerFat**Choices**

Ham Sub on Wheat, ½ sub 4
Ham Sub on White, ½ sub........................ 5
Roast Beef Sub on Wheat, ½ sub........... 4
Roast Beef Sub on White, ½ sub............ 5
Turkey Breast Sub on Wheat, ½ sub 4
Turkey Breast Sub on White, ½ sub 4
Vegetarian Sub, 8-inch............................. 4

Salads

Chef Salad (without cheese), with lite salad dressing, 1 7

Some Low-*POINT* Ideas

each

½ Ham Sub on Wheat
½ Roast Beef Sub on Wheat
½ Turkey Breast Sub on Wheat
½ Turkey Breast Sub on White
8-inch Vegetarian Sub

each

½ Ham Sub on White
½ Roast Beef Sub on White

1 Chef Salad (without cheese) with lite salad dressing

KFC®

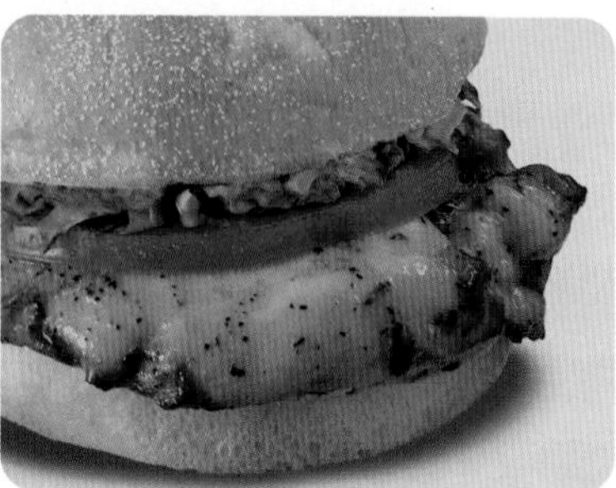

KFC Original Recipe® Chicken

Breast, 1 (with skin removed by customer) 3
Breast, 1 (as served with skin) 10
Drumstick, 1 (as served with skin) 4
Thigh, 1 (as served with skin) 6
Whole Wing, 1 (as served with skin) 4

KFC Extra Crispy™ Chicken

Breast, 1 (as served with skin) 12
Drumstick, 1 (as served with skin) 5
Thigh, 1 (as served with skin) 10
Whole Wing, 1 (as served with skin) 5

KFC Hot & Spicy Chicken

Breast, 1 (as served with skin) 12
Drumstick, 1 (as served with skin) 4
Thigh, 1 (as served with skin) 9
Whole Wing, 1 (as served with skin) 5

POINTS

Wings

Honey BBQ Wings Pieces, 6 pieces 15
Hot Wings™ Pieces, 6 pieces 12

Sandwiches

Honey BBQ Flavored Chicken Sandwich, with sauce, 1 6
Original Recipe® Chicken Sandwich, with sauce, 1 10
Original Recipe® Chicken Sandwich, without sauce, 1 8
Tender Roast® Chicken Sandwich, with sauce, 1 8
Tender Roast® Chicken Sandwich, without sauce, 1 6
Triple Crunch® Chicken Sandwich, with sauce, 1 13
Triple Crunch® Chicken Sandwich, without sauce, 1 9
Triple Crunch® Zinger Chicken Sandwich, with sauce, 1 13
Triple Crunch® Zinger Chicken Sandwich, without sauce, 1 9

Crispy Strips

Colonel's Crispy Strips®, 3 pieces 7
Spicy Crispy Strips, 3 pieces 8

Popcorn Chicken

Popcorn Chicken, 1 small serving 9
Popcorn Chicken, 1 large serving 16

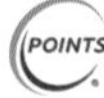

PotPie

Chunky Chicken Pot Pie, 1 18

SideItems

BBQ Baked Beans, 1 serving 3
Biscuit, 1 4
Cole Slaw, 1 serving 5
Corn on the Cob, 1 3
Macaroni & Cheese, 1 serving 4
Mashed Potatoes with Gravy, 1 serving 3
Potato Salad, 1 serving 5
Potato Wedges, 1 serving 6

Cake

Double Chocolate Chip Cake, 1 serving 8

Colonel's™Pies

Apple Pie, 1 slice 7
Pecan Pie, 1 slice 11
Strawberry Creme Pie, 1 slice 6

LittleBucket™Parfaits

Chocolate Cream, 1 7
Fudge Brownie, 1 6
Lemon Creme, 1 9
Strawberry Shortcake, 1 4

MealIdeas

1 KFC Original Recipe® Chicken Drumstick (with skin)
1 Biscuit

1 Honey BBQ Flavored Chicken Sandwich (with sauce)
1 serving Corn on the Cob

1 Tender Roast® Chicken Sandwich (without sauce)
1 Strawberry Shortcake Little Bucket™ Parfait

Krispy Kreme Doughnuts®

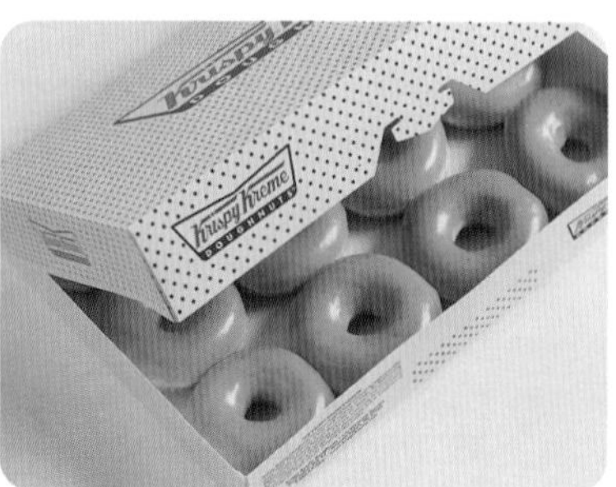

YeastDoughnuts

Krispy Kreme Original Glazed Doughnut, 1 5
Cinnamon Twist, 1 5
Fudge Iced Glazed Doughnut, 1 7
Fudge Iced with Sprinkles, 1 5
Maple Iced Glazed Doughnut, 1 4

FilledYeast**Doughnuts**

Cinnamon Apple Filled Doughnut, 1 6
Fudge Iced Creme Filled Doughnut, 1 8
Fudge Iced Custard Filled Doughnut, 1 7
Glazed Creme Filled Doughnut, 1 8
Glazed Lemon Filled Doughnut, 1 7
Glazed Raspberry Filled Doughnut, 1 6
Powdered Blueberry Filled Doughnut, 1 6

POINTS

CakeDoughnuts

Traditional Cake Doughnut, 1 5
Fudge Iced Cake Doughnut, 1 5
Glazed Blueberry Doughnut, 1 7
Glazed Devil's Food Doughnut, 1 9

CinnamonBun**&**Crullers

Cinnamon Bun, 1 5
Glazed Cruller, 1 6
Fudge Iced Glazed Cruller, 1 6

Some Low-*POINT* Ideas

1 Maple Iced Glazed Yeast Doughnut

each

1 Krispy Kreme Original Glazed Yeast Doughnut
1 Traditional Cake Doughnut
1 Cinnamon Twist
1 Fudge Iced Cake Doughnut
1 Cinnamon Bun

each

1 Cinnamon Apple Filled Yeast Doughnut
1 Glazed Raspberry Filled Yeast Doughnut
1 Powdered Blueberry Filled Yeast Doughnut
1 Glazed Cruller
1 Fudge Iced Glazed Cruller

Krystal®

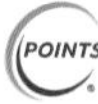

Burgers&Sandwiches

THE FAMOUS KRYSTAL®, 1 4
CHEESE KRYSTAL®, 1 4
DOUBLE KRYSTAL®, 1 6
DOUBLE CHEESE KRYSTAL®, 1 7
Bacon Cheese Krystal, 1 4
Krystal Chik Sandwich, 1 5
PLAIN PUP®, 1 4
CORN PUP®, 1 7
CHILI CHEESE PUP®, 1 5

Chili

Krystal Chili, 1 serving 4

Fries

Regular Fries, 1 serving 8
Chili Cheese Fries, 1 serving 12

Breakfast

Plain Biscuit, 1 6
Sausage Biscuit, 1 11
Chik Biscuit, 1 8
Bacon, Egg & Cheese Biscuit, 1 9
KRYSTAL SUNRISER®, 1 6
Country Breakfast, 1 serving 16
Hash Browns, 1 serving 4

Desserts&Shakes

Apple Turnover, 1 serving 5
Chocolate Shake, 1 serving 9
Lemon Meringue Pie, 1 serving 8

MealIdeas

1 PLAIN PUP®
1 serving Krystal Chili

1 CHEESE KRYSTAL®
1 serving Apple Turnover

1 KRYSTAL SUNRISER®
1 serving Hash Browns

Little Caesars® Pizza

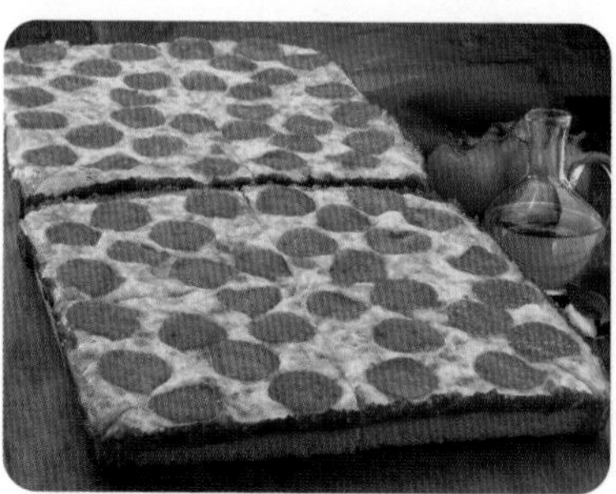

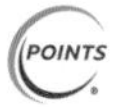

12-inch Medium Round Pizza

Cheese Pizza, 1 slice (⅛ of 12-inch pizza) 4

Pepperoni Pizza, 1 slice (⅛ of 12-inch pizza) 4

14-inch Large Round Pizza

Cheese Pizza, 1 slice (1/10 of 14-inch pizza) 4

Meatsa® Pizza, 1 slice (1/10 of 14-inch pizza) 6

Pepperoni Pizza, 1 slice (1/10 of 14-inch pizza) 5

Supreme Pizza, 1 slice (1/10 of 14-inch pizza) 6

Veggie!Veggie!® Pizza, 1 slice (1/10 of 14-inch pizza) 4

16-inch Extra Large Round Pizza

Cheese Pizza, 1 slice (1/12 of 16-inch pizza) 4

Pepperoni Pizza, 1 slice (1/12 of 16-inch pizza) 5

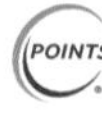

12-inch Medium Deep Dish Pizza

Cheese Pizza, 1 slice (⅛ of 12-inch pizza) 5

Pepperoni Pizza, 1 slice (⅛ of 12-inch pizza) 5

12-inch Thin Crust Pizza

Cheese, 1 slice (⅛ of 12-inch pizza) 3

Pepperoni, 1 slice (⅛ of 12-inch pizza) 3

14-inch Large Deep Dish Pizza

Cheese Pizza, 1 slice (⅛ of 14-inch pizza) 6

Pepperoni Pizza, 1 slice (⅛ of 14-inch pizza) 7

14-inch Thin Crust Pizza

Cheese, 1 slice (1/10 of 14-inch pizza) 3

Pepperoni, 1 slice (1/10 of 14-inch pizza) 4

Pizza by the Slice

Cheese Pizza, 1 slice (⅙ of 14-inch pizza) 6

Pepperoni Pizza, 1 slice (⅙ of 14-inch pizza) 8

Cold Sandwiches

Deli Ham & Cheese, 1 13

Deli Italian, 1 16

Deli Veggie, 1 17

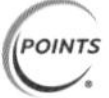

BabyPan!Pan!® CinnamonCrazyStick& ItalianCheese Bread®

Baby Pan! Pan!®, 1 pizza 9
Cinnamon Crazy Stick, 1 1
Italian Cheese Bread®, 1 piece 3

CrazyBread®&CrazySauce®

Crazy Bread®, 1 slice 2
Crazy Sauce®, ½ cup 0

Salads (without dressing)

Antipasto Salad, 1 4
Tossed Side Salad, 1 1

SaladDressings

Fat Free Italian Dressing, 1 packet (3 Tbsp) 0
Italian Dressing, 1 packet (3 Tbsp) 6
Ranch Dressing, 1 packet (3 Tbsp) 6

MealIdeas

1 Antipasto Salad with
 1 packet Fat Free Italian Dressing
1 slice Crazy Bread® with
 ½ cup Crazy Sauce®

2 slices of 12-inch Thin Crust
 Cheese Pizza
1 Tossed Side Salad with
 1 packet Fat Free Italian Dressing

1 Baby Pan!Pan!® Pizza
1 Tossed Side Salad with
 1 packet Fat Free Italian Dressing

Long John Silver's®

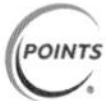

Fish, Seafood, & Chicken

Baked Cod with Glaze, 1 piece 15
Battered-Dipped Chicken, 1 piece..........3
Battered-Dipped Fish, 1 piece 6
Battered-Dipped Shrimp, 1 piece 1
Breaded Clams, 1 serving 6
Crunchy Shrimp, 28 pieces......................10

Meal

Baked Cod Meal (1 piece of glazed cod, rice, coleslaw, and corn cobbette without butter), 1 serving...22

Sandwiches

Chicken Sandwich, 1 7
Fish Sandwich, 1.......................................10
Ultimate Fish Sandwich®, 1..................11

Side Items

Cheese Sticks, 3 3
Clam Chowder, 1 bowl 5
Coleslaw, 1 serving 5
Corn Cobbette, 1 1
Corn Cobbette, with butter, 1.................3
Crumblies®, 1 serving 4
Fries, 1 regular serving 5
Hushpuppy, 1 piece 1
Rice, 1 serving..3

Desserts

Chocolate Creme Pie, 1 8
Pecan Pie, 1 8
Pineapple Creme Pie, 1............................7

Meal Ideas

4 pieces Batter-Dipped Shrimp
1 Corn Cobbette

1 bowl Clam Chowder
3 Cheese Sticks

2 pieces Batter-Dipped Chicken
3 Cheese Sticks

MAZZIO'S®

POINTS

Appetizers

Breadstick, 1 ... 2
Cheese Dippers, 4 slices (¼ serving) ... 7
Cheese Nachos, ½ serving ... 9
Cinnamon Sticks, 4 (¼ serving) ... 8
Meat Nachos, ½ serving ... 12
Wings of Fire, with sauce, 4 (¼ large serving) ... 10
Wings of Fire, with sauce, 4 (½ small serving) ... 9

Original Crust Pizza

"Mazzio's Works" Pizza, 1 slice (⅛ of medium pizza) ... 6
California Alfredo Pizza, 1 slice (⅛ of medium pizza) ... 6
Cheese Pizza, 1 slice (⅛ of medium pizza) ... 4
Chicken Club Pizza, 1 slice (⅛ of medium pizza) ... 5
Combo Pizza, 1 slice (⅛ of medium pizza) ... 5
Meatbuster® Pizza, 1 slice (⅛ of medium pizza) ... 6
Mexican Pizza, 1 slice (⅛ of medium pizza) ... 8
Pepperoni Pizza, 1 slice (⅛ of medium pizza) ... 5
Sausage Pizza, 1 slice (⅛ of medium pizza) ... 5
Supremebuster® Pizza, 1 slice (⅛ of medium pizza) ... 5

POINTS

Deep Pan Pizza

"Mazzio's Works" Pizza, 1 slice (⅛ of medium pizza) ... 9
California Alfredo Pizza, 1 slice (⅛ of medium pizza) ... 9
Cheese Pizza, 1 slice (⅛ of medium pizza) ... 7
Chicken Club Pizza, 1 slice (⅛ of medium pizza) ... 8
Combo Pizza, 1 slice (⅛ of medium pizza) ... 8
Meatbuster® Pizza, 1 slice (⅛ of medium pizza) ... 9
Mexican Pizza, 1 slice (⅛ of medium pizza) ... 10
Pepperoni Pizza, 1 slice (⅛ of medium pizza) ... 7
Sausage Pizza, 1 slice (⅛ of medium pizza) ... 8
Supremebuster® Pizza, 1 slice (⅛ of medium pizza) ... 8

Pizzeria Crust Pizza

"Mazzio's Works" Pizza, 1 slice (⅛ of large pizza) ... 9
California Alfredo Pizza, 1 slice (⅛ of large pizza) ... 9
Cheese Pizza, 1 slice (⅛ of large pizza) ... 7
Chicken Club Pizza, 1 slice (⅛ of large pizza) ... 8
Combo Pizza, 1 slice (⅛ of large pizza) ... 8
Meatbuster® Pizza, 1 slice (⅛ of large pizza) ... 9

POINTS

Mexican Pizza, 1 slice (⅛ of large pizza) 11

Pepperoni Pizza, 1 slice (⅛ of medium pizza) 7

Sausage Pizza, 1 slice (⅛ of large pizza) 9

Supremebuster® Pizza, 1 slice (⅛ of large pizza) 8

ThinCrustPizza

"Mazzio's Works" Pizza, 1 slice (⅛ of medium pizza) 5

California Alfredo Pizza, 1 slice (⅛ of medium pizza) 5

Cheese Pizza, 1 slice (⅛ of medium pizza) 4

Chicken Club Pizza, 1 slice (⅛ of medium pizza) 4

Combo Pizza, 1 slice (⅛ of medium pizza) 5

Meatbuster® Pizza, 1 slice (⅛ of medium pizza) 5

Mexican Pizza, 1 slice (⅛ of medium pizza) 6

Pepperoni Pizza, 1 slice (⅛ of medium pizza) 4

Sausage Pizza, 1 slice (⅛ of medium pizza) 4

Supremebuster® Pizza, 1 slice (⅛ of medium pizza) 4

POINTS

Pasta

Fettuccine Alfredo, 1 serving 29

Italian Sampler, 1 serving 37

Lasagna with Meat Sauce, 1 serving 16

Spaghetti with Marinara, 1 serving 19

Spaghetti with Meat Sauce, 1 serving 26

Spaghetti with Meatballs, 1 serving 35

Calzones

Ham-Bacon-Cheddar Calzone, 1 slice (1/10 of calzone) 6

Pepperoni Calzone, 1 slice (1/10 of calzone) 5

Some Low-*POINT* Ideas

1 Breadstick

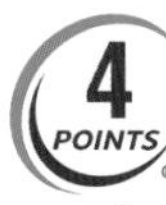

each

1 slice of medium Original Crust Cheese Pizza
1 slice of medium Thin Crust Cheese Pizza
1 slice of medium Thin Crust Pepperoni or Sausage Pizza
1 slice of medium Thin Crust Supremebuster® Pizza

each

1 slice of medium Original Crust Chicken Club Pizza
1 slice of medium Original or Thin Crust Combo Pizza
1 slice of medium Thin Crust "Mazzio's Works" Pizza
1 slice of Pepperoni Calzone

McDonald's®

POINTS

Sandwiches

Hamburger, 1 ... 6
Cheeseburger, 1 ... 7
Quarter Pounder®, 1 ... 10
Quarter Pounder® with Cheese, 1 ... 13
Big Mac®, 1 ... 14
Big N' Tasty® with Cheese, 1 ... 14
Big N' Tasty®, 1 ... 13
Chicken McGrill®, 1 ... 9
Chicken McGrill®, without mayonnaise, 1 ... 6
Crispy Chicken Sandwich, 1 ... 12
Filet-O-Fish®, 1 ... 11

French Fries

French Fries, 1 small serving ... 5
French Fries, 1 medium serving ... 10
French Fries, 1 large serving ... 12
Super Size® French Fries, 1 serving ... 14
McValue French Fries, 1 serving ... 7

Chicken McNuggets®/Sauces

Chicken McNuggets®, 4 pieces ... 5
Chicken McNuggets®, 6 pieces ... 7
Chicken McNuggets®, 9 pieces ... 11
Barbecue Sauce, 1 packet ... 1
Honey Mustard, 1 packet ... 1
Honey, 1 packet ... 1
Hot Mustard, 1 packet ... 1
Light Mayonnaise, 1 packet ... 1
Sweet 'N Sour Sauce, 1 packet ... 1

Salads & Salad Dressings

Bacon Ranch Crispy Chicken Salad, 1 serving ... 9
Bacon Ranch Grilled Chicken Salad, 1 serving ... 6
Bacon Ranch Salad, 1 serving ... 3
Caesar Salad, 1 serving ... 2
California Cobb Salad, 1 serving ... 4
Crispy Chicken Caesar Salad, 1 serving ... 7
Crispy Chicken California Cobb Salad, 1 serving ... 9
Grilled Chicken Caesar Salad, 1 serving ... 4
Grilled Chicken California Cobb Salad, 1 serving ... 6
Newman's Own California Cobb Dressing, 1 pouch ... 2
Newman's Own Creamy Caesar Dressing – Restaurant Style, 1 pouch ... 5
Newman's Own Light Balsamic Vinaigrette Dressing, 1 pouch ... 2
Newman's Own Ranch Dressing – Restaurant Style, 1 pouch ... 8

Breakfast

English Muffin, 1 ... 3
Egg McMuffin®, 1 ... 7
Sausage McMuffin®, 1 ... 9
Sausage McMuffin® with Egg, 1 ... 11
Bacon, Egg & Cheese Biscuit, 1 ... 12
Biscuit, 1 ... 6
Ham, Egg & Cheese Bagel, 1 ... 13
Hash Browns, 1 serving ... 3
Hotcakes, with 2 pats margarine and 1 packet syrup, 1 serving ... 13
Hotcakes, without syrup & margarine, 1 serving ... 7

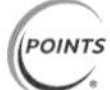

Sausage Biscuit with Egg, 1 12
Sausage Biscuit, 1 10
Sausage Breakfast Burrito, 1 7
Sausage, 1 5
Scrambled Eggs, 1 serving (2 eggs) 4
Spanish Omelete Bagel, 1 16
Steak, Egg & Cheese Bagel, 1 17

Muffin, Danish & Roll

Apple Danish, 1 8
Cheese Danish, 1 9
Cinnamon Roll, 1 9

Desserts & Shakes

Baked Apple Pie, 1 6
Butterfinger® McFlurry™, 1 14
Chocolate Chip Cookie, 1 serving 7
Chocolate Shake, 16 oz 13
Fruit 'n Yogurt Parfait (without granola), 1 3
Hot Caramel Sundae, 1 8
Hot Fudge Sundae, 1 8
M&M® McFlurry™, 1 14
McDonaldland® Cookies, 1 package 5
Nestle Crunch® McFlurry™, 1 14
Nuts (for sundaes), 1 serving 1
Oreo® McFlurry™, 1 13
Snack Size Fruit 'n Yogurt Parfait, 1 3
Strawberry Shake, 16 oz 13
Strawberry Sundae, 1 6
Vanilla Reduced Fat Ice Cream Cone, 1 3
Vanilla Shake, 16 oz 13

Meal Ideas

4-piece Chicken McNuggets®
1 Vanilla Reduced Fat Ice Cream Cone

1 Chicken McGrill® (without mayonnaise)
1 small serving French Fries

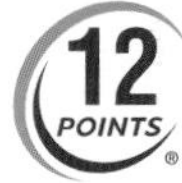

1 Cheeseburger
1 small serving French Fries

Monical's Pizza®

POINTS

Starters

Breadsticks (plain), 1 stick 4
Cheddar Cheese, 1 serving 3
Cheddar Nuggets (without sauce), 4 pieces 3
Hot Wings (without ranch), 3 pieces 5
Nacho Cheese, 1 serving 4
Pepperollies (without marinara), 3 ... 29
Plain Mild Cheddar Cheese Fries (with toppings), 1 pound 31
Plain Mild Cheddar Cheese Fries (without toppings), 1 pound 26
Plain Nacho Cheese Fries (with toppings), 1 pound 34
Plain Nacho Cheese Fries (without toppings), 1 pound 29
Tomato Sauce, 1 serving 1

Monical'sPizza®

(7" Thick Crust)

BBQ Chicken, 1 whole 28
Cheese Free, 1 whole 15
Cheese, 1 whole 21
Delight, 1 whole 24
Deluxe, 1 whole 25
Happy Heart, 1 whole 16
Italian Special, 1 whole 39
Pepperoni, 1 whole 24
Sausage, 1 whole 21
Veggie, 1 whole 26

POINTS

Monical'sPizza®

(8" Thick Crust)

BBQ Chicken, 1 whole 24
Cheese Free, 1 whole 11
Cheese, 1 whole 16
Delight, 1 whole 20
Deluxe, 1 whole 21
Happy Heart, 1 whole 15
Italian Special, 1 whole 35
Pepperoni, 1 whole 20
Sausage, 1 whole 17
Veggie, 1 whole 22

Pasta

4 Cheese Lasagna, 1 individual serving 14
Garlic Stick, 2 8
Meatballs, 3 6
Ravioli, 1 individual serving 10
Spaghetti, 1 individual serving 9
Supreme Blend of Cheese, 1 serving 3
Tortellini, 1 individual serving 8

Sandwiches (without chips)

BBQ Chicken, 8" sub 17
Classic Sub, 8" sub 23
Ham & Cheese, 8" sub 25
Hot Sicilian, 8" sub 23
Italian Beef, 8" sub 14
Meatball, 8" sub 26
Turkey, 8" sub 13

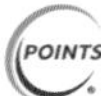

Salads

Chef Salad, 1 9
Individual Salad, 1 2

Dressings

1000 Island, 2 Tbsp 4
Creamy Italian Lite, 2 Tbsp 1
Creamy Italian, 2 Tbsp 3
Fat Free Vinaigrette, 2 Tbsp 0
Monical's® Sweet & Tart, 2 Tbsp 7
Ranch, 2 Tbsp 4

MealIdeas

1 Individual Salad with
2 Tbsp Fat Free Vinaigrette Dressing
4 pieces Cheddar Nuggets with
1 serving Tomato Sauce

1 Individual Salad with
2 Tbsp Creamy Italian Lite Dressing
3 pieces Hot Wings (without ranch)

1 Chef Salad with
2 Tbsp Fat Free Vinaigrette Dressing
1 Plain Breadstick

Mr. Goodcents®

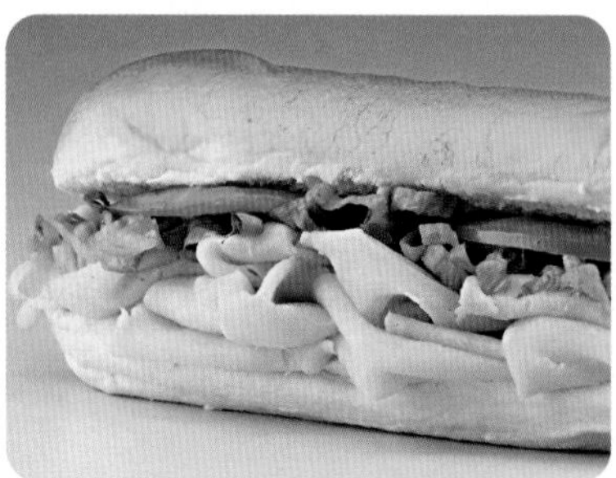

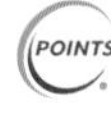

Sandwiches

Centsable Sub™ on Wheat, ½ sandwich (7¾") 11
Cheese Mix on Wheat, ½ sandwich (7¾") 15
Chicken Parmesan on Wheat, ½ sandwich (7¾") 9
Chicken Salad on Wheat, ½ sandwich (7¾") 10
Ham and Cheese on Wheat, ½ sandwich (7¾") 10
Italian on Wheat, ½ sandwich (7¾") 15
Meatball on Wheat, ½ sandwich (7¾") 17
Mr. Goodcents Original™ on Wheat, ½ sandwich (7¾") 13
Mr. Goodcents Steak Alfredo on Wheat, ½ sandwich (7¾") 11
Penny Club™ on Wheat, ½ sandwich (7¾") 9
Pepperoni and Cheese on Wheat, ½ sandwich (7¾") 17
Roast Beef on Wheat, ½ sandwich (7¾") 10
Salami on Wheat, ½ sandwich (7¾") 16
Sausage on Wheat, ½ sandwich (7¾") 15
Seafood Salad on Wheat, ½ sandwich (7¾") 12
Tuna Salad on Wheat, ½ sandwich (7¾") 13
Turkey on Wheat, ½ sandwich (7¾") 9
Veggie on Wheat, ½ sandwich (7¾") 7

Salads

California Pasta Salad, 1 2
Chef's Salad, 1 2
Chicken Salad on Garden Salad, 1 5
Country Potato Salad, 1 4

Meals

Chicken Alfredo Mostiaccioli and Bread Stick Centsational Size, 1 serving 15
Chicken Parmesan Mostiaccioli and Bread Stick, 1 serving 10
Chicken Parmesan Mostiaccioli Centsational Size with Bread Stick, 1 serving 14
Kids Mostiaccioli with Red Sauce and Grilled Chicken Strips, 1 serving 6
Lasagna and Breadstick, 1 serving 14
Mostiaccioli Alfredo and Bread Stick, 1 serving 12

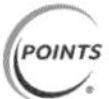

Mostiaccioli with Red Sauce and Bread Stick Centsational™ Size, 1 serving 11

Quarter with Roast Beef and Chicken Noodle Soup, 1 serving (¼ sandwich and 8 oz soup) 10

Soup

Chicken Noodle Soup with Crackers, 1 serving 6

Golden Broccoli Cheese Soup, 1 serving 8

Breadsticks

Bread Stick, 1 2

Cookies

Chocolate Chip Cookie, 1 11

Peanut Butter Cookie, 1 8

MealIdeas

1 Chef's Salad
1 Bread Stick

1 Chicken Salad on Garden Salad
1 Bread Stick

½ Veggie on Wheat Sandwich
1 California Pasta Salad

Mrs. Fields®

POINTS

Cookies

Butter Cookie, 1 7
Butter Toffee Cookie, 1 7
Chewy Chocolate Fudge Cookie, 1 7
Coconut Macadamia Cookie, 1 6
Debra's Special Cookie, 1 6
Milk Chocolate Chip Cookie with Walnuts, 1 8
Milk Chocolate Chip Cookie, 1 6
Milk Chocolate Chip Macadamia Cookie, 1 8
Oatmeal Raisin Cookie, 1 5
Peanut Butter Cookie, 1 7
Pumpkin Harvest Cookie, 1 6
Semi-Sweet Chocolate Chip Cookie with Pecans, 1 7
Semi-Sweet Chocolate Chip Cookie with Walnuts, 1 7
Semi-Sweet Chocolate Chip Cookie, 1 7
Triple Chocolate Cookie, 1 7
White Chunk Macadamia Cookie, 1 7

CookieNibbler™

Butter Cookie Nibbler™, 2 3
Chewy Chocolate Fudge Cookie Nibbler™, 2 2
Debra's Special Cookie Nibbler™, 2 2
Milk Chocolate Chip Cookie Nibbler™, 2 2
Milk Chocolate Chip with Walnuts Cookie Nibbler™, 2 3
Peanut Butter Cookie Nibbler™, 2 3
Semi-Sweet Chocolate Chip Cookie Nibbler™, 2 2
Semi-Sweet Chocolate Chip with Walnuts Cookie Nibbler™, 2 3
White Chunk Macadamia Cookie Nibbler™, 2 3

Muffins

Banana Walnut Muffin, 1 9
Blueberry Muffin, 1 9
Chocolate Chip Muffin, 1 10
Mandarin Orange Muffin, 1 10

Bagels (without spread)

Cinnamon Raisin Bagel, 1 5
Everything Bagel, 1 5
Onion Bagel, 1 5
Plain Bagel, 1 5
Poppyseed Bagel, 1 5
Sesame Bagel, 1 5

Brownies&Bar

Double Fudge Brownie, 1 9
Fudge Walnut Brownie, 1 12
Pecan Fudge Brownie, 1 9
Pecan Pie Brownie, 1 9
Peanut Butter Dream Bar, 1 18

Some Low-*POINT* Ideas

each

2 Chewy Chocolate Fudge Cookie Nibbler™
2 Debra's Special Cookie Nibbler™
2 Milk Chocolate Chip Cookie Nibbler™
2 Semi-Sweet Chocolate Chip Cookie Nibbler™

each

2 Butter Cookie Nibbler™
2 Semi-Sweet or Milk Chocolate Chip with Walnuts Cookie Nibbler™
2 Peanut Butter Cookie Nibbler™
2 White Chunk Macadamia Cookie Nibbler™

each

1 Oatmeal Raisin Cookie
1 Cinnamon Raisin, Everything, Onion, Plain, Poppyseed, or Sesame Bagel (without spread)

PAPA JOHN'S®

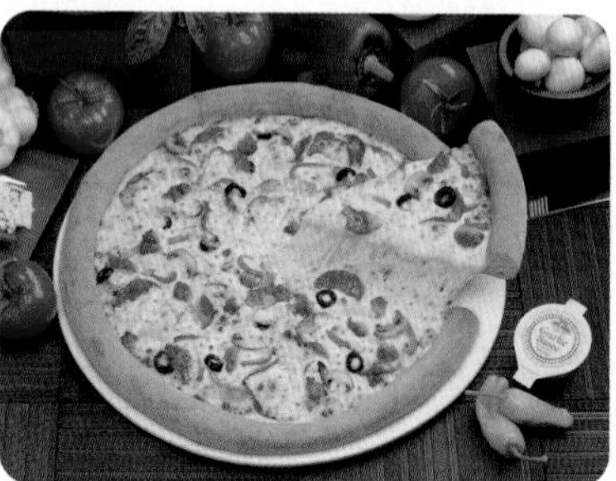

OriginalCrust**Pizza**

(14-inch Large Pizza)

	POINTS
All the Meats™ Pizza, 1 slice (⅛ of large pizza)	9
Cheese Pizza, 1 slice (⅛ of large pizza)	6
Garden Special™ Pizza, 1 slice (⅛ of large pizza)	6
Pepperoni Pizza, 1 slice (⅛ of large pizza)	7
Sausage Pizza, 1 slice (⅛ of large pizza)	7
The Works™ Pizza, 1 slice (⅛ of large pizza)	8

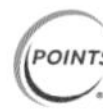

ThinCrust**Pizza**

(14-inch Large Pizza)

	POINTS
All the Meats™ Pizza, 1 slice (⅛ of large pizza)	10
Cheese Pizza, 1 slice (⅛ of large pizza)	5
Garden Special™ Pizza, 1 slice (⅛ of large pizza)	5
Pepperoni Pizza, 1 slice (⅛ of large pizza)	6
Sausage Pizza, 1 slice (⅛ of large pizza)	7
The Works™ Pizza, 1 slice (⅛ of large pizza)	8

BreadStick**&**Cheese**Sticks**

Bread Stick, 1	3
Cheese Sticks, 2	4

Some Low-*POINT* Ideas

1 Bread Stick

2 Cheese Sticks

each

1 slice of large Thin Crust Cheese Pizza
1 slice of large Thin Crust Garden Special™ Pizza

Papa Murphy's®
TAKE 'N' BAKE PIZZA

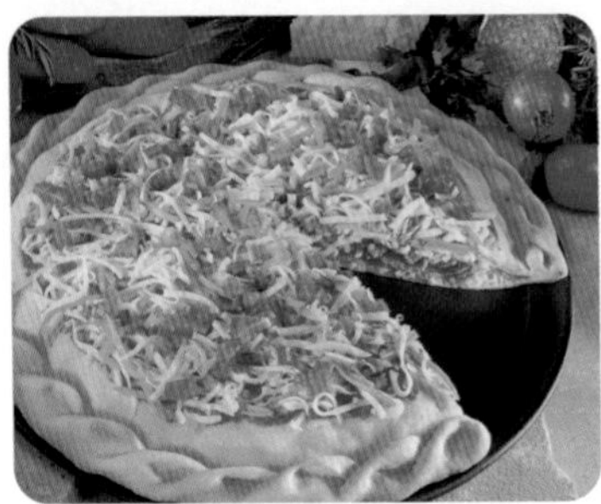

Pizza

Cheese Pizza, 1 slice (1⁄12 of family size pizza) 6

Chicago-Style Stuffed Pizza™, 1 slice (1⁄12 of family size pizza) 11

Chicken & Bacon Stuffed Pizza™, 1 slice (1⁄12 of family size pizza) 10

Hawaiian Pizza™, 1 slice (1⁄12 of family size pizza) 7

Murphy's Combo™ Pizza, 1 slice (1⁄12 of family size pizza) 8

Pepperoni Pizza, 1 slice (1⁄12 of family size pizza) 7

Perfect Pizza, 1 slice (1⁄12 of family size pizza) 7

Sausage Pizza, 1 slice (1⁄12 of family size pizza) 6

The Rancher Pizza, 1 slice (1⁄12 of family size pizza) 8

The Vegetarian Pizza, 1 slice (1⁄12 of family size pizza) 7

Some Low-*POINT* Ideas

each

1 slice of family size Cheese Pizza
1 slice of family size Sausage Pizza

each

1 slice of family size Hawaiian Pizza™
1 slice of family size Pepperoni Pizza
1 slice of family size Perfect Pizza
1 slice of family size The Vegetarian Pizza

each

1 slice of family size Murphy's Combo™ Pizza
1 slice of family size The Rancher Pizza

Pickerman's Soups & Sandwiches

POINTS

Sandwiches (includes bread, meat and vegetable; cheese, dressing, or sauce may be added)

B.L.T., 1 7
BBQ, 1 8
Caesar Salad, 1 10
Chicken Caesar, 1 11
Chicken, 1 6
Classic Club, 1 8
Garden Salad, 1 9
Greek Salad, 1 10
Ham & Swiss, 1 8
Meatball, 1 14
Numero Uno, 1 9
Roast Beef, 1 7
That's Italian, 1 9
Tuna, 1 8
Turkey, 1 6
Veggie, 1 5

Soup

5 Star Mushroom, 1 serving 3
Asiago Cheese Bisque, 1 serving 6
Beef Noodle, 1 serving 2
Black Bean, 1 serving 3
Black Forest Lentil, 1 serving 1
Broccoli Cheddar, 1 serving 5
Cauliflower Cheddar, 1 serving 5
Chicken Gumbo, 1 serving 2
Chicken Noodle, 1 serving 2
Chicken with Rice, 1 serving 4
Clam Chowder, 1 serving 4
Country Bean, 1 serving 2
Country Potato, 1 serving 3
Country Vegetable, 1 serving 1
French Onion, 1 serving 1
Loaded Baked Potato, 1 serving 5
Minestrone, 1 serving 1
Pickerman's Stew, 1 serving 4
Potato Cheddar, 1 serving 5
Potato Cream Cheese, 1 serving 4
Roasted Garlic Tomato, 1 serving 5
Santa Fe Tortilla, 1 serving 3
Southwest Roasted Corn, 1 serving 2
Spring Asparagus, 1 serving 4
Texas Chili, 1 serving 4
Tomato Basil, 1 serving 1
Vegetable Beef Barley, 1 serving 2
Vegetarian Chili, 1 serving 3
White Chicken Chili, 1 serving 3
Wisconsin Cheese, 1 serving 4

Cheese, Dressing & Sauce

Light Cream Cheese, 1 serving 2
Provolone, 1 oz 3
Swiss, 1 oz 3
Italian Dressing, 1 Tbsp 6
Salad Dressing, 1 Tbsp 2
Mayo, 1 Tbsp 3

MealIdeas

1 serving Black Forest Lentil Soup
1 Veggie Sandwich (without cheese, dressing, or sauce)

1 serving French Onion Soup
1 Veggie Sandwich with 1 oz Swiss Cheese (without dressing or sauce)

1 serving Tomato Basil Soup
1 Chicken Sandwich with 1 Tbsp Mayo (without cheese or dressing)

Pizza Hut®

POINTS

Thin'NCrispy® pizza

Beef Topping Pizza, 1 slice (1/8 of medium pizza) ... 6

Beef Topping Pizza, 1 slice (1/12 of large pizza) ... 6

Cheese Only Pizza, 1 slice (1/8 of medium pizza) ... 5

Cheese Only Pizza, 1 slice (1/12 of large pizza) ... 4

Chicken Supreme Pizza, 1 slice (1/8 of medium pizza) ... 4

Chicken Supreme Pizza, 1 slice (1/12 of large pizza) ... 4

Diced Chicken Pizza, 1 slice (1/8 of medium pizza) ... 5

Diced Chicken Pizza, 1 slice (1/12 of large pizza) ... 4

Italian Sausage Pizza, 1 slice (1/8 of medium pizza) ... 7

Italian Sausage Pizza, 1 slice (1/12 of large pizza) ... 6

Meat Lover's® pizza, 1 slice (1/8 of medium pizza) ... 7

Meat Lover's® pizza, 1 slice (1/12 of large pizza) ... 7

Pepperoni Lover's® pizza, 1 slice (1/8 of medium pizza) ... 6

Pepperoni Lover's® pizza, 1 slice (1/12 of large pizza) ... 6

Pepperoni Pizza, 1 slice (1/8 of medium pizza) ... 5

Pepperoni Pizza, 1 slice (1/12 of large pizza) ... 5

Pork Topping Pizza, 1 slice (1/8 of medium pizza) ... 6

POINTS

Pork Topping Pizza, 1 slice (1/12 of large pizza) ... 6

Quartered Ham Pizza, 1 slice (1/8 of medium pizza) ... 4

Quartered Ham Pizza, 1 slice (1/12 of large pizza) ... 4

Sausage Lover's® pizza, 1 slice (1/8 of medium pizza) ... 8

Sausage Lover's® pizza, 1 slice (1/12 of large pizza) ... 7

Super Supreme Pizza, 1 slice (1/8 of medium pizza) ... 6

Super Supreme Pizza, 1 slice (1/12 of large pizza) ... 6

Supreme Pizza, 1 slice (1/8 of medium pizza) ... 6

Supreme Pizza, 1 slice (1/12 of large pizza) ... 5

Veggie Lover's® pizza, 1 slice (1/8 of medium pizza) ... 4

Veggie Lover's® pizza, 1 slice (1/12 of large pizza) ... 4

PanPizza

Beef Topping Pizza, 1 slice (1/8 of medium pizza) ... 7

Beef Topping Pizza, 1 slice (1/12 of large pizza) ... 7

Cheese Only Pizza, 1 slice (1/8 of medium pizza) ... 7

Cheese Only Pizza, 1 slice (1/12 of large pizza) ... 7

Chicken Supreme Pizza, 1 slice (1/8 of medium pizza) ... 6

Chicken Supreme Pizza, 1 slice (1/12 of large pizza) ... 6

POINTS

Diced Chicken Pizza, 1 slice (⅛ of medium pizza) 6

Diced Chicken Pizza, 1 slice (1/12 of large pizza) 6

Italian Sausage Pizza, 1 slice (⅛ of medium pizza) 8

Italian Sausage Pizza, 1 slice (1/12 of large pizza) 8

Meat Lover's® pizza, 1 slice (⅛ of medium pizza) 8

Meat Lover's® pizza, 1 slice (1/12 of large pizza) 8

Pepperoni Lover's® pizza, 1 slice (⅛ of medium pizza) 8

Pepperoni Lover's® pizza, 1 slice (1/12 of large pizza) 8

Pepperoni Pizza, 1 slice (⅛ of medium pizza) 7

Pepperoni Pizza, 1 slice (1/12 of large pizza) 7

Pork Topping Pizza, 1 slice (⅛ of medium pizza) 7

Pork Topping Pizza, 1 slice (1/12 of large pizza) 7

Quartered Ham Pizza, 1 slice (⅛ of medium pizza) 6

Quartered Ham Pizza, 1 slice (1/12 of large pizza) 6

Sausage Lover's® pizza, 1 slice (⅛ of medium pizza) 9

Sausage Lover's® pizza, 1 slice (1/12 of large pizza) 9

Super Supreme Pizza, 1 slice (⅛ of medium pizza) 8

Super Supreme Pizza, 1 slice (1/12 of large pizza) 8

POINTS

Supreme Pizza, 1 slice (⅛ of medium pizza) 7

Supreme Pizza, 1 slice (1/12 of large pizza) 7

Veggie Lover's® pizza,1 slice (⅛ of medium pizza) 6

Veggie Lover's® pizza, 1 slice (1/12 of large pizza) 5

Hand-Tossed Style Pizza

Beef Topping Pizza, 1 slice (⅛ of medium pizza) 6

Beef Topping Pizza, 1 slice (1/12 of large pizza) 6

Cheese Only Pizza, 1 slice (⅛ of medium pizza) 5

Cheese Only Pizza, 1 slice (1/12 of large pizza) 5

Chicken Supreme Pizza, 1 slice (⅛ of medium pizza) 5

Chicken Supreme Pizza, 1 slice (1/12 of large pizza) 4

Diced Chicken Pizza, 1 slice (⅛ of medium pizza) 5

Diced Chicken Pizza, 1 slice (1/12 of large pizza) 5

Italian Sausage Pizza, 1 slice (⅛ of medium pizza) 7

Italian Sausage Pizza, 1 slice (1/12 of large pizza) 6

Meat Lover's® pizza, 1 slice (⅛ of medium pizza) 7

Meat Lover's® pizza, 1 slice (1/12 of large pizza) 7

Pepperoni Lover's® pizza, 1 slice (⅛ of medium pizza) 7

Hand-Tossed Style Pizza (con't)

POINTS

Pepperoni Lover's® pizza, 1 slice (1/12 of large pizza) 6

Pepperoni Pizza, 1 slice (1/8 of medium pizza) 5

Pepperoni Pizza, 1 slice (1/12 of large pizza) 5

Pork Topping Pizza, 1 slice (1/8 of medium pizza) 6

Pork Topping Pizza, 1 slice (1/12 of large pizza) 5

Quartered Ham Pizza, 1 slice (1/8 of medium pizza) 5

Quartered Ham Pizza, 1 slice (1/12 of large pizza) 4

Sausage Lover's® pizza, 1 slice (1/8 of medium pizza) 8

Sausage Lover's® pizza, 1 slice (1/12 of large pizza) 7

Super Supreme Pizza, 1 slice (1/8 of medium pizza) 6

Super Supreme Pizza, 1 slice (1/12 of large pizza) 6

Supreme Pizza, 1 slice (1/8 of medium pizza) 6

Supreme Pizza, 1 slice (1/12 of large pizza) 5

Veggie Lover's® pizza, 1 slice (1/8 of medium pizza) 5

Veggie Lover's® pizza, 1 slice (1/12 of large pizza) 4

StuffedCrustPizza

Beef Topping Pizza, 1 slice (1/12 of large pizza) 10

Cheese Only Pizza, 1 slice (1/12 of large pizza) 9

POINTS

Chicken Supreme Pizza, 1 slice (1/12 of large pizza) 8

Diced Chicken Pizza, 1 slice (1/12 of large pizza) 9

Italian Sausage Pizza, 1 slice (1/12 of large pizza) 11

Meat Lovers® pizza, 1 slice (1/12 of large pizza) 11

Pepperoni Lover's® pizza, 1 slice (1/12 of large pizza) 11

Pepperoni Pizza, 1 slice (1/12 of large pizza) 9

Pork Topping Pizza, 1 slice (1/12 of large pizza) 10

Quartered Ham Pizza, 1 slice (1/12 of large pizza) 8

Sausage Lover's® pizza, 1 slice (1/12 of large pizza) 11

Super Supreme Pizza, 1 slice (1/12 of large pizza) 11

Supreme Pizza, 1 slice (1/12 of large pizza) 10

Veggie Lover's® pizza, 1 slice (1/12 of large pizza) 8

TheBigNewYorkerPizza

Beef Topping Pizza, 1 slice (1/8 of 16-inch pizza) 11

Cheese Only Pizza, 1 slice (1/8 of 16-inch pizza) 9

Chicken Supreme Pizza, 1 slice (1/8 of 16-inch pizza) 9

Diced Chicken Pizza, 1 slice (1/8 of 16-inch pizza) 9

Italian Sausage Pizza, 1 slice (1/8 of 16-inch pizza) 12

POINTS

Meat Lover's® pizza, 1 slice (⅛ of 16-inch pizza) 13
Pepperoni Lover's® pizza, 1 slice (⅛ of 16-inch pizza) 12
Pepperoni Pizza, 1 slice (⅛ of 16-inch pizza) 9
Pork Topping Pizza, 1 slice (⅛ of 16-inch pizza) 11
Quartered Ham Pizza, 1 slice (⅛ of 16-inch pizza) 8
Sausage Lover's® pizza, 1 slice (⅛ of 16-inch pizza) 14
Super Supreme Pizza, 1 slice (⅛ of 16-inch pizza) 12
Supreme Pizza, 1 slice (⅛ of 16-inch pizza) 11
Veggie Lover's® pizza, 1 slice (⅛ of 16-inch pizza) 8

ChicagoDishPizza

Beef Topping Pizza, 1 slice (⅛ pizza) 10
Cheese Only Pizza, 1 slice (⅛ pizza) 9
Chicken Supreme Pizza, 1 slice (⅛ pizza) 8
Diced Chicken Pizza, 1 slice (⅛ pizza) 9
Italian Sausage Pizza, 1 slice (⅛ pizza) 10
Meat Lover's® pizza, 1 slice (⅛ pizza) 11
Pepperoni Lover's® pizza, 1 slice (⅛ pizza) 10
Pepperoni Pizza, 1 slice (⅛ pizza) 9
Pork Topping Pizza, 1 slice (⅛ pizza) 10

POINTS

Quartered Ham Pizza, 1 slice (⅛ pizza) 8
Sausage Lover's® pizza, 1 slice (⅛ pizza) 10
Super Supreme Pizza, 1 slice (⅛ pizza) 10
Supreme Pizza, 1 slice (⅛ pizza) 9
Veggie Lover's® pizza, 1 slice (⅛ pizza) 8

PersonalPanPizza

Beef Topping Pizza, 1 slice 4
Cheese Only Pizza, 1 slice 3
Chicken Supreme Pizza, 1 slice 3
Diced Chicken Pizza, 1 slice 3
Italian Sausage Pizza, 1 slice 4
Meat Lover's® pizza, 1 slice 4
Pepperoni Pizza, 1 slice 3
Pork Topping Pizza, 1 slice 4
Quartered Ham Pizza, 1 slice 3
Pepperoni Lover's® pizza, 1 slice 4
Sausage Lover's® pizza, 1 slice 4
Super Supreme Pizza, 1 slice 4
Supreme Pizza, 1 slice 4
Veggie Lover's® pizza, 1 slice 3

Appetizers&Bread

Bread Sticks, 1 serving 3
Garlic Bread, 1 slice 4
Hot Buffalo Wings, 2 pieces 3
Mild Buffalo Wings, 2 pieces 3
Cheese Breadsticks, 1 5
Cheese Garlic Bread, 1 6
Chicken Munchers, 2 pieces 2

Pizza Hut®

Appetizers & Breads (con't)

Jalapeno Poppers, 2 pieces 3
Mozzarella Sticks, 2 pieces 3
Onion Rings, ¼ serving 4
Bread Stick Dipping Sauce, 1 serving 1
Wing Blue Cheese Dipping Sauce, 1½ oz 7
Wing Ranch Dipping Sauce, 1½ oz 6

Salad Dressings

Caesar Dressing, 2 Tbsp 4
French Dressing, 2 Tbsp 4
Italian Dressing, 2 Tbsp 4
Lite Italian Dressing, 2 Tbsp 2
Lite Ranch Dressing, 2 Tbsp 2
Ranch Dressing, 2 Tbsp 3
Thousand Island Dressing, 2 Tbsp 3

Pasta

CAVATINI® pasta, 1 serving 9
CAVATINI SUPREME® pasta, 1 serving 10
Pasta Bakes® marinara with meatballs, 1 serving 24
Pasta Bakes® marinara, 1 serving 19
Pasta Bakes® primavera with chicken, 1 serving 24
Pasta Bakes® primavera, 1 serving 22
Spaghetti with Marinara Sauce, 1 serving 10
Spaghetti with Meat Sauce, 1 serving 14
Spaghetti with Meatballs, 1 serving 13

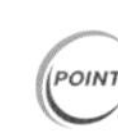

Desserts

Apple Dessert Pizza, 1 slice 5
Cherry Dessert Pizza, 1 slice 5
Cinnamon Sticks, 2 pieces 4
White Icing Dipping Cup, 1 4

Some Low-*POINT* Ideas

2 pieces Chicken Munchers

each

1 slice Cheese Only Personal Pan Pizza
1 slice Chicken Supreme Personal Pan Pizza
1 slice Pepperoni Personal Pan Pizza
1 serving Veggie Lover's® personal pan pizza
2 pieces Jalapeno Poppers
2 pieces Mozzarella Sticks

each

1 slice Cheese Only Large Thin 'N Crispy® pizza
1 slice Quartered Ham Medium or Large Thin 'N Crispy® pizza
1 slice Veggie Lover's® Medium or Large Thin 'N Crispy® pizza
1 slice Beef Topping Personal Pan Pizza
1 slice Pepperoni Lover's® personal pan pizza

Planet Smoothie

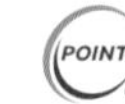

Smoothies (all smoothies are 22 fl oz, except for Captain Kid, which is 12 fl oz)

Item	POINTS
Berry Bada-Bing™, 1	6
Big Bang™, 1	6
Billy Bob Banana™, 1	6
Captain Kid, 1	4
Chocolate Chimp™, 1	7
Chocolate Elvis™, 1	10
Frozen Goat™, 1	7
Grape Ape™, 1	6
Hangover Over™, 1	6
Leapin' Lizard™, 1	4
Lunar Lemonade (Raspberry)™, 1	7
Lunar Lemonade™, 1	7
Mediterranean Monster™, 1	5
Merlin's Pineapple Lean Body, 1	8
Merlin's Pineapple Myoplex, 1	8
Merlin's Strawberry Lean Body, 1	9
Merlin's Strawberry MyoPlex, 1	9
Mr. Mongo-Chocolate™, 1	10
Mr. Mongo-Strawberry™, 1	8
PBJ™, 1	12
Rasmanian Devil™, 1	5
Road Runner™, 1	5
Screamsicle™, 1	7
Shag-a-delic™, 1	8
Spazz™, 1	5
The Last Mango™, 1	7
Thelma & Louise™, 1	4
Twig & Berries™, 1	5
Two Piece Bikini-Chocolate™, 1	6
Two Piece Bikini-Strawberry™, 1	5
Vinnie Del Rocco™, 1	7
Werewolf™, 1	4
Yo' Adriane™, 1	5
Zeus Juice™, 1	4

Some Low-*POINT* Ideas

each

12 fl oz Captain Kid Smoothie
22 fl oz Leapin' Lizard™ Smoothie
22 fl oz Thelma & Louise™ Smoothie
22 fl oz Werewolf™ Smoothie
22 fl oz Zeus Juice™ Smoothie

each

22 fl oz Mediterranean Monster™ Smoothie
22 fl oz Rasmanian Devil™ Smoothie
22 fl oz Road Runner™ Smoothie
22 fl oz Twig & Berries™ Smoothie
22 fl oz Two Piece Bikini-Strawberry™ Smoothie

each

22 fl oz Berry Bada-Bing™ Smoothie
22 fl oz Big Bang™ Smoothie
22 fl oz Billy Bob Banana™ Smoothie
22 fl oz Grape Ape™ Smoothie
22 fl oz Two Piece Bikini-Chocolate™ Smoothie

Pretzel Time®

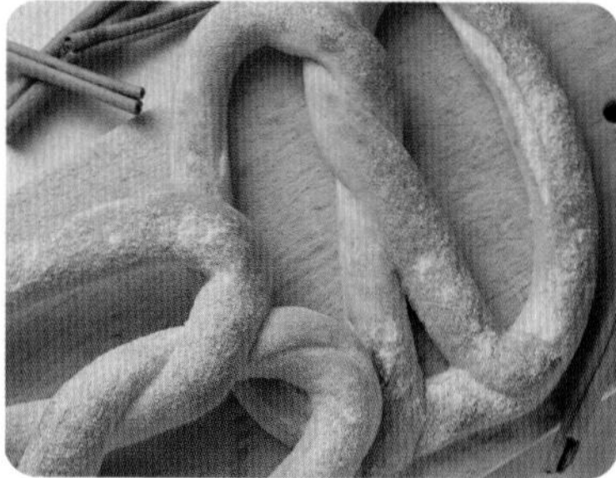

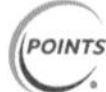

Pretzels

Plain Pretzel, without butter, 1 6
Regular Pretzel, with butter, 1 7
Cinnamon Sugar Pretzel, 1 7
Garlic Pretzel, 1 7
Parmesan Pretzel, 1 7
Sour Cream & Onion Pretzel, 1 7
Whole Wheat Pretzel, without butter, 1 5
Whole Wheat Pretzel, with butter, 1 ...6

Some Low-*POINT* Ideas

1 Whole Wheat Pretzel (without butter)

each

1 Plain Pretzel (without butter)
1 Whole Wheat Pretzel (with butter)

each

1 Regular Pretzel (with butter)
1 Cinnamon Sugar Pretzel
1 Garlic Pretzel
1 Parmesan Pretzel
1 Sour Cream & Onion Pretzel

Round Table® Pizza

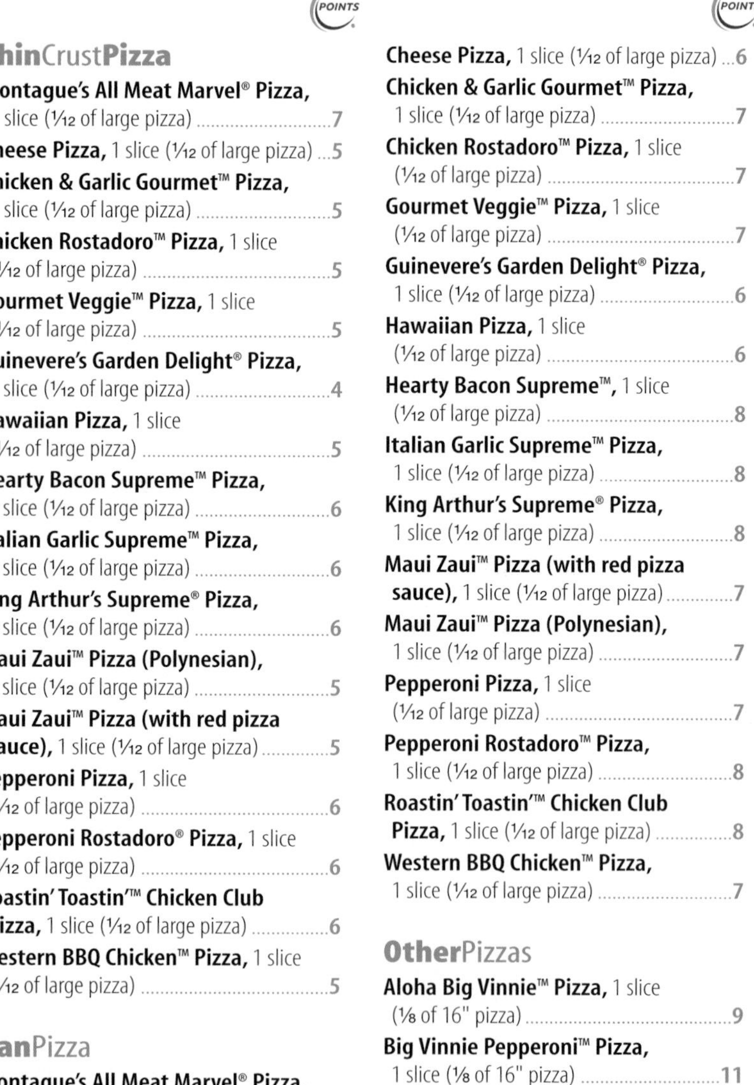

POINTS

ThinCrustPizza

Montague's All Meat Marvel® Pizza, 1 slice (1⁄12 of large pizza) 7

Cheese Pizza, 1 slice (1⁄12 of large pizza) ... 5

Chicken & Garlic Gourmet™ Pizza, 1 slice (1⁄12 of large pizza) 5

Chicken Rostadoro™ Pizza, 1 slice (1⁄12 of large pizza) 5

Gourmet Veggie™ Pizza, 1 slice (1⁄12 of large pizza) 5

Guinevere's Garden Delight® Pizza, 1 slice (1⁄12 of large pizza) 4

Hawaiian Pizza, 1 slice (1⁄12 of large pizza) 5

Hearty Bacon Supreme™ Pizza, 1 slice (1⁄12 of large pizza) 6

Italian Garlic Supreme™ Pizza, 1 slice (1⁄12 of large pizza) 6

King Arthur's Supreme® Pizza, 1 slice (1⁄12 of large pizza) 6

Maui Zaui™ Pizza (Polynesian), 1 slice (1⁄12 of large pizza) 5

Maui Zaui™ Pizza (with red pizza sauce), 1 slice (1⁄12 of large pizza) 5

Pepperoni Pizza, 1 slice (1⁄12 of large pizza) 6

Pepperoni Rostadoro® Pizza, 1 slice (1⁄12 of large pizza) 6

Roastin' Toastin'™ Chicken Club Pizza, 1 slice (1⁄12 of large pizza) 6

Western BBQ Chicken™ Pizza, 1 slice (1⁄12 of large pizza) 5

PanPizza

Montague's All Meat Marvel® Pizza, 1 slice (1⁄12 of large pizza) 8

POINTS

Cheese Pizza, 1 slice (1⁄12 of large pizza) ... 6

Chicken & Garlic Gourmet™ Pizza, 1 slice (1⁄12 of large pizza) 7

Chicken Rostadoro™ Pizza, 1 slice (1⁄12 of large pizza) 7

Gourmet Veggie™ Pizza, 1 slice (1⁄12 of large pizza) 7

Guinevere's Garden Delight® Pizza, 1 slice (1⁄12 of large pizza) 6

Hawaiian Pizza, 1 slice (1⁄12 of large pizza) 6

Hearty Bacon Supreme™, 1 slice (1⁄12 of large pizza) 8

Italian Garlic Supreme™ Pizza, 1 slice (1⁄12 of large pizza) 8

King Arthur's Supreme® Pizza, 1 slice (1⁄12 of large pizza) 8

Maui Zaui™ Pizza (with red pizza sauce), 1 slice (1⁄12 of large pizza) 7

Maui Zaui™ Pizza (Polynesian), 1 slice (1⁄12 of large pizza) 7

Pepperoni Pizza, 1 slice (1⁄12 of large pizza) 7

Pepperoni Rostadoro™ Pizza, 1 slice (1⁄12 of large pizza) 8

Roastin' Toastin'™ Chicken Club Pizza, 1 slice (1⁄12 of large pizza) 8

Western BBQ Chicken™ Pizza, 1 slice (1⁄12 of large pizza) 7

OtherPizzas

Aloha Big Vinnie™ Pizza, 1 slice (1⁄8 of 16" pizza) 9

Big Vinnie Pepperoni™ Pizza, 1 slice (1⁄8 of 16" pizza) 11

Some Low-*POINT* Ideas

1 slice of large Thin Crust Guinevere's Garden Delight® Pizza

each

1 slice of large Thin Crust Cheese Pizza
1 slice of large Thin Crust Maui Zaui™ (Polynesian or with red pizza sauce) Pizza
1 slice of large Thin Crust Western BBQ Chicken™ Pizza

each

1 slice of large Thin Crust Hearty Bacon Supreme™ Pizza
1 slice of large Thin Crust King Arthur's Supreme® Pizza
1 slice of large Thin Crust Pepperoni Rostadoro® Pizza

Ryan's® Grill, Buffet & Bakery®

POINTS®

Foods Available on the Mega Bar® Buffet

MainCourses

Alaskan Salmon, 1 serving....5
Baked Fish, 1 serving....2
Chicken Breast, 1 serving....5
Chicken Livers, 1 cup....5
Chicken Pot Pie, 1 cup....3
Fettucini Noodles, 1 cup....8
Grilled Ham, 1 serving....4
Meatloaf, 1 serving....6
Meatloaf Patties, 1 serving....8
Mexican Style Beef Casserole, 1 cup...11
Petite Sirloin, 1 serving....6
Sausage, Sliced in Peppers and Onions, 1 cup....7
Sausage, Sliced in Saurkraut, 1 cup....6
Sauteed Mushrooms, ½ cup....0
Sauteed Onions, ½ cup....0
Sauteed Peppers and Onions, ½ cup....0
Sirloin Tips, Plain, 1 serving....5
Nacho Cheese Sauce, ¼ cup....2
Shredded Taco Cheese, ½ cup....12
Spaghetti Noodles, 1 cup....8
Spaghetti Sauce with Meatballs, ½ cup....1
Taco Meat, 1 cup....4
Vegetable Lasagna, 1 cup....9

SideItems

Ambrosia Salad, ½ cup....1
Bowtie Pasta and Vegetables, 1 cup....3
Breaded Okra, ¾ cup....1
Breaded Sweet Potato Nuggets, 7....2
Broccoli and Cauliflower Salad, 1 cup...3
Broccoli Spears, 1 cup....0
Brussel Sprouts, 1 cup....1
Cabbage, 1 cup....1
Candied Sweet Potatoes with Marshmallows, 1 cup....2
Corn on the Cob, 1 ear....1
Corn, ½ cup....1
Country Cookin' Fresh Sweet Potatoes, 1 cup....4
Glazed Baby Carrots with Sauce, ½ cup....2
Great Northern Beans, 1 cup....1
Green Beans, 1 cup....1
Lima Beans and Corn, 1 cup....3
Lima Beans, ⅔ cup....2
Macaroni & Cheese, 1 cup....8
Mashed Potatoes, 1 cup....2
Mexican Rice, 1 cup....4
Pasta Salad with Broccoli & Vegetable Blend, 1 cup....3
Pea Salad, 1 cup....4
Peas and Carrots, 1 cup....1
Pinto Beans, 1 cup....1
Seafood Pasta Salad, 1 cup....3
Seasoned Red Bliss Potatoes, 1 cup....4
Sliced Carrots, 1 cup....0
Stewed Tomatoes with Yellow Squash, 1 cup....0
Turnip Greens, 1 cup....1
Yellow Squash, 1 cup....2

POINTS

Soups

Clam Chowder, 1 cup 4
Vegetable Beef Soup, 1 cup 2

Salads & Salad Dressings

Blackeye Pea Salad, 1 cup 1
Chicken Salad, ⅓ cup 5
Corn Salad, 1 cup 3
Crab Salad, ½ cup 2
Low Fat Cottage Cheese, ½ cup 2
Marinated Seven Bean Salad, ⅓ cup 2
Seafood AuGratin, 1 cup 2
Tomato and Onion Salad, 1 cup 1
Blue Cheese Dressing, ⅓ cup 4
Fat Free Ranch Dressing, 2 Tbsp 1
French Dressing, 1 serving 3
Golden Italian Dressing, 1 serving 4
Ranch Dressing, 1 serving 4
Thousand Island Dressing, 1 serving 3

Breads

Cinnamon Butter, 1 15
Country Cornbread Muffins, 1 7
Country Mexican Cornbread, 1 5
Yeast Roll, 1 7

Desserts

Apple Cobbler, ½ cup 6
Blackberry Cobbler, ½ cup 6
Blueberry Cobbler, ½ cup 6
Cherry Cobbler, ½ cup 6
Chocolate Chip Cookies, 1 6

POINTS

Chocolate Soft Serve, ½ cup 3
No Fat No Sugar Added Butter Pecan Frozen Yogurt, ½ cup 2
Old Fashioned Fudge Topping, 2 Tbsp 3
Peach Cobbler, ½ cup 6
Peanut Butter Cookies, 1 3
Raisin Oatmeal Cookies, 1 2
Ranger Cookies, 1 3
Sugar Cookies, 1 3
Sugar Free Chocolate Pudding, ½ cup 2
Sugar Free Cookies, 2 3
Sugar Free Gelatin, ½ cup 0
Sugar Free Whip Topping, 2 Tbsp 0

*Known as Fire Mountain® Grill Buffet Restaurant in select markets.

Meal Ideas

1 cup Vegetable Beef Soup
1 serving Baked Fish
½ cup Sauteed Peppers and Onions
½ cup Sugar Free Gelatin

1 cup Tomato and Onion Salad
1 cup Chicken Pot Pie
½ cup Sugar Free Chocolate Pudding with 2 tbsp Sugar Free Whipped Topping

1 serving Grilled Ham
1 cup Candied Sweet Potatoes with Marshmallows
1 cup Broccoli Spears
½ cup No Fat No Sugar Added Butter Pecan Frozen Yogurt

Schlotzsky's® Deli

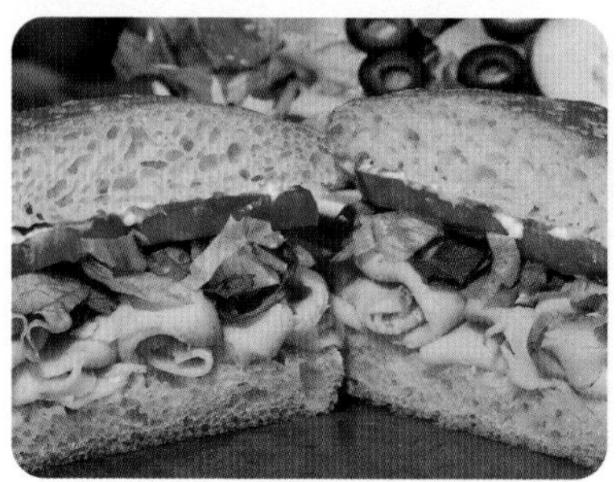

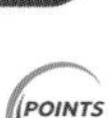

Schlotzsky's® Deli Light Menu - 7 Grams of Fat or Less

5Sandwicheswith7Grams ofFatorLess

Chicken Breast, 1 small ... 6
Dijon Chicken, 1 small ... 6
Pesto Chicken, 1 small ... 7
Smoked Turkey Breast, 1 small ... 7
The Vegetarian, 1 small ... 7

Wrapwith7GramsofFatorLess

Asian Almond Chicken, 1 ... 9

7Saladswith7GramsofFator Less (without dressing, croutons or chow mein noodles)

Caesar Salad, 1 ... 3
Chicken Caesar Salad, 1 ... 5
Chinese Chicken Salad, 1 ... 4
Fruit Salad, 1 small ... 1
Fruit Salad, 1 regular ... 2

POINTS

Garden Salad, 1 small ... 0
Garden Salad, 1 regular ... 0

10Soupswith7GramsofFat orLess

Chicken Gumbo Soup, 1 cup ... 2
Chicken Tortilla Soup, 1 cup ... 3
Gourmet Vegetable Beef Soup, 1 cup ... 2
Minestrone Soup, 1 cup ... 1
Monterrey Black Bean Soup, 1 cup ... 4
Old-Fashioned Chicken Noodle Soup, 1 cup ... 2
Ravioli Soup, 1 cup ... 2
Red Beans & Rice Soup, 1 cup ... 3
Timberline Chili, 1 cup ... 4
Vegetarian Vegetable Soup, 1 cup ... 2

Sandwiches

BLT, 1 small ... 8
Chicken Club, 1 small ... 10
Corned Beef, 1 small ... 8
Corned Beef Reuben, 1 small ... 12
Fiesta Chicken, 1 small ... 13
Ham & Cheese Original, 1 small ... 11
Pastrami & Swiss, 1 small ... 13
Pastrami Reuben, 1 small ... 14
Roast Beef, 1 small ... 9
Roast Beef & Cheese, 1 small ... 13
Santa Fe Chicken, 1 small ... 8
Texas Schlotzsky's®, 1 small ... 12
The Original, 1 small ... 12
The Philly, 1 small ... 13
Turkey & Bacon Club, 1 small ... 13
Turkey Guacamole, 1 small ... 9

POINTS

Turkey Original, 1 small 13
Turkey Reuben, 1 small 12
Vegetable Club, 1 small 8
Western Vegetarian, 1 small 10

Wraps

Chicken Caesar, 1 12
Salsa Chicken with Cheddar, 1 10

8-inch Sourdough Crust Pizza

Bacon, Tomato & Mushroom Pizza, 1 whole 13
Barbeque Chicken Pizza, 1 whole 15
Chicken & Pesto Pizza, 1 whole 14
Double Cheese & Pepperoni Pizza, 1 whole 16
Double Cheese Pizza, 1 whole 12
Fresh Tomato & Pesto Pizza, 1 whole ... 11
Mediterranean Pizza, 1 whole 11
Smoked Turkey & Jalapeño Pizza, 1 whole 13
Thai Chicken Pizza, 1 whole 14
The Original Combination Pizza, 1 whole 14
Tuscan Herb Pizza, 1 whole 11
Vegetarian Special Pizza, 1 whole 12

Salads (without dressing, croutons, or chow mein noodles)

Chicken Salad, 1 regular 8
Greek Salad, 1 3
Ham & Turkey Chef's Salad, 1 4
Smoked Turkey Chef's Salad, 1 4
Chow Mein Noodles, 1 packet 2
Garlic Cheese Croutons, 1 packet 1

POINTS

Salad Dressings

Greek Balsamic Vinaigrette, 1 packet (3 Tbsp) 5
Light Italian Dressing, 1 packet (3 Tbsp) 2
Light Spicy Ranch Dressing, 1 packet (3 Tbsp) 4
Olde World Caesar Dressing, 1 packet (3 Tbsp) 6
Sesame Ginger Vinaigrette, 1 packet (3 Tbsp) 5
Spicy Ranch Dressing, 1 packet (3 Tbsp) 7
Thousand Island Dressing, 1 packet (3 Tbsp) 6
Traditional Ranch Dressing, 1 packet (3 Tbsp) 8

Soups

Boston Clam Chowder, 1 cup 6
Broccoli Cheese with Florets Soup, 1 cup 6
Chicken with Wild Rice Soup, 1 cup 9
Pilgrim Corn Chowder, 1 cup 7
Potato with Bacon Soup, 1 cup 5
Tuscan Tomato Basil Soup, 1 cup 8
Wisconsin Cheese Soup, 1 cup 8

Schlotzsky's® Deli-Style Potato Chips

Baked Chips (regular), 1 individual bag (1 oz) 2
Potato Chips (regular or flavored), 1 individual bag (1.5 oz) 5

Desserts

Chocolate Chip Cookie, 1 4
Cookies & Creme Cheesecake, 1 serving 8
Cookies with Real M&M's®, 1 3
Cranberry Walnut Crunch Cookie, 1 4
Fudge Brownie Cake, 1 serving 10
Fudge Chocolate Chip Cookie, 1 4
Golden Raisin Oatmeal Cookie, 1 4
New York Creamstyle Cheesecake, 1 serving 8
Oatmeal Raisin Cookie, 1 3
Peanut Butter Cookie, 1 4
Strawberry Swirl Cheesecake, 1 serving 7
Sugar Cookie, 1 4
Triple Chocolate Chip Cookie, ½ 4
White Chocolate Macadamia Cookie, ½ 4

Kid's Deals (without cookie or 12 oz. soft drink)

Cheese Pizza, 1 10
Cheese Sandwich, 1 9
Ham & Cheese Sandwich, 1 10
PBJ Sandwich, 1 10
Pepperoni Pizza, 1 11
Turkey & Cheese Sandwich, 1 9

MealIdeas

1 small Deli Light Chicken Breast Sandwich
1 regular Deli Light Garden Salad with 1 packet Light Italian Dressing

1 cup Deli Light Minestrone Soup
1 Deli Light Chicken Caesar Salad
1 Oatmeal Raisin Cookie

1 cup Deli Light Minestrone Soup
1 small Santa Fe Chicken Sandwich
1 individual bag Regular Baked Chips

Sizzler®

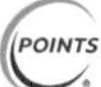

Entrees (without choice of starch and cheese toast)

Coho Salmon without Sizzling Veggies, 1 serving 9

Coho Salmon with Sizzling Veggies, 1 serving 9

Grilled Cajun Chicken Sandwich, 1 19

Grilled Chicken Club Sandwich, 1 20

Ribeye Steak, 14 oz 28

Sizzlin' Garlic Herb Chicken without Grilled Mushrooms and Onions, 1 serving 6

Sizzlin' Garlic Herb Chicken with Grilled Onions and Mushrooms, 1 serving 10

Sizzlin' Grilled Shrimp Skewers without Sizzling Vegetables, 2 skewers 5

Sizzlin' Grilled Shrimp Skewers with Sizzling Veggies (without Melted Margarine), 1 serving (2 skewers with veggies) 6

Steak & Grilled Shrimp Skewers with Sizzling Veggies (with Melted Margarine), 1 serving (2 skewers with veggies) 8

Steak & Hibachi Chicken, 1 serving 11

Steak & Lobster Tail (without Melted Margarine), 1 serving 12

Steak & Shrimp Scampi, 1 serving 12

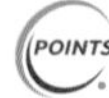

Some Low-*POINT* Ideas

2 Sizzlin' Grilled Shrimp Skewers (without sizzling vegetables)

each

1 serving Sizzlin' Garlic Herb Chicken (without grilled mushrooms and onions)

1 serving Sizzlin' Grilled Shrimp Skewers with Sizzling Veggies (without melted margarine)

1 serving Steak & Grilled Shrimp Skewers with Sizzling Veggies (without melted margarine)

SMOOTHIE KING®

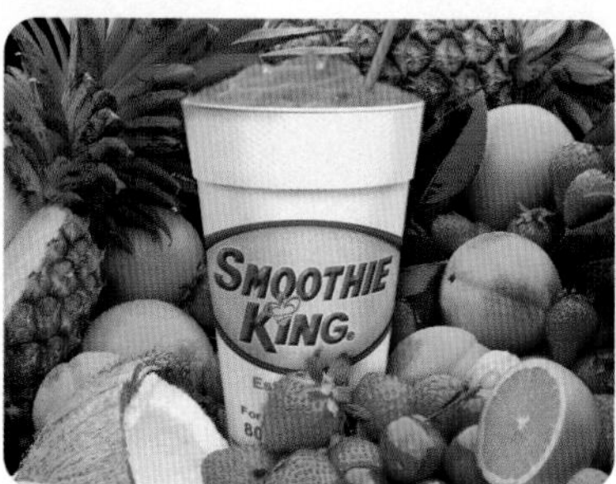

POINTS

Smoothie (20 oz serving)

Amaretto, 1 serving 2
Angel Food™, 1 serving 6
Banana Boat™, 1 serving 11
Blackberry Dream™, 1 serving 6
Blueberry Heaven™, 1 serving 5
Caribbean Way™, 1 serving 7
Celestial Cherry High™, 1 serving 5
Cherry Picker™, 1 serving 7
Coconut Surprise™, 1 serving 9
Cranberry Cooler™, 1 serving 10
Cranberry Supreme™, 1 serving 11
French Roast, 1 serving 3
French Vanilla, 1 serving 2
Grape Expectations™, 1 serving 8
Grape Expectations II™, 1 serving 10
Hazelnut, 1 serving 2
Hearty Apple™, 1 serving 7
High Protein - Almond Mocha, 1 serving 8
High Protein - Banana, 1 serving 9

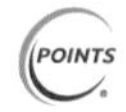

High Protein - Chocolate, 1 serving 8
High Protein - Lemon, 1 serving 8
High Protein - Pineapple, 1 serving 8
Hulk™ - Chocolate, 1 serving 19
Hulk™ - Strawberry, 1 serving 21
Hulk™ - Vanilla, 1 serving 19
Immune Builder™, 1 serving 6
Instant Vigor™, 1 serving 7
Irish Crème, 1 serving 2
Island Treat®, 1 serving 6
Lemon Twist Banana®, 1 serving 6
Lemon Twist Strawberry®, 1 serving 8
Light & Fluffy®, 1 serving 7
Malt, 1 serving 21
MangoFest™, 1 serving 6
Mo cuccino™, 1 serving 9
Mocha, 1 serving 4
Muscle Punch®, 1 serving 6
Muscle Punch Plus™, 1 serving 6
Orange Ka-Bam™, 1 serving 6
Peach Slice™, 1 serving 6
Peach Slice Plus™, 1 serving 9
Peanut Power®, 1 serving 11
Peanut Power Plus™ Grape, 1 serving 15
Peanut Power Plus™ Strawberry, 1 serving 14
Pep Upper®, 1 serving 6
Pina Colada Island™, 1 serving 11
Pineapple Pleasure, 1 serving 6
Pineapple Surf™, 1 serving 8
Power Punch™, 1 serving 8

POINTS

Power Punch Plus®, 1 serving 9
Raspberry Sunrise™, 1 serving 6
Shake, 1 serving 21
Slim & Trim™ - Chocolate, 1 serving 5
Slim & Trim™ - Orange-Vanilla, 1 serving 4
Slim & Trim™ - Strawberry, 1 serving 7
Slim & Trim™ - Vanilla, 1 serving 4
Strawberry Kiwi Breeze™, 1 serving 6
Strawberry X-Treme™, 1 serving 7
Super Punch™, 1 serving 8
Super Punch Plus®, 1 serving 10
The Activator® - Chocolate, 1 serving 8
The Activator® - Strawberry, 1 serving 10
The Activator® - Vanilla, 1 serving 8
Yogurt D-Lite™, 1 serving 7
Youth Fountain™, 1 serving 5

HeaterZ™ High Protein Hot Smoothie Brews (12 oz serving)

Amaretto, 1 serving 3
Banana Nut, 1 serving 8
Blueberry Muffin, 1 serving 7
Chocolate Peanut Butter Cup, 1 serving 8
Cinnamon Oatmeal Raisin, 1 serving 8
Coconut, 1 serving 9
French Roast, 1 serving 3
French Vanilla, 1 serving 3
Hazelnut, 1 serving 3
Irish Crème, 1 serving 3
Mocha, 1 serving 5

POINTS

KingStix™

Apple Cinnamon, 1 7
Bavarian Plain, 1 7
Blueberry Turnover, 1 8
Cheddar Jalapeno, 1 9
Pizza, 1 8
Spinach Feta, 1 8

Iced Coffee

Amaretto, 1 serving 3
French Roast, 1 serving 3
French Vanilla, 1 serving 3
Hazelnut, 1 serving 3
Irish Crème, 1 serving 3
Mocha, 1 serving 4

Hot Coffee

Amaretto, 1 serving 3
French Roast, 1 serving 3
French Vanilla, 1 serving 3
Hazelnut, 1 serving 3
Irish Crème, 1 serving 3
Mocha, 1 serving 4

Kid's Kups (12 oz serving)

Berry Interesting™, 1 serving 3
Choc-A-Laka™, 1 serving 4
Gimme-Grape™, 1 serving 3
Smarti Tarti™, 1 serving 3

Some Low-*POINT* Ideas

each

1 serving Amaretto Smoothie
1 serving Hazelnut Smoothie
1 serving Irish Crème Smoothie

each

1 serving French Roast Smoothie
1 serving Amaretto, French Vanilla, or Irish Crème HeaterZ™ High Protein Hot Smoothie Brew
1 serving Amaretto, French Roast, or Hazelnut Iced Coffee
1 serving French Vanilla, Hazelnut, or Irish Crème Hot Coffee
1 serving Berry Interesting™, Gimme-Grape™, or Smarti-Tarti™ Kid's Kup

each

1 serving Mocha Smoothie
1 serving Slim & Trim™ Orange-Vanilla or Vanilla Smoothie
1 serving Mocha Iced Coffee

Sonic®, America's Drive-In®

POINTS

Burgers

No. 1 Sonic® Burger, 1 14
No. 1 Sonic® Cheeseburger, 1 16
No. 2 Sonic® Burger, 1 11
No. 2 Sonic® Cheeseburger, 1 13
Sonic® Bacon Cheeseburger, 1 18
***Super*Sonic™ No. 1,** 1 24
***Super*Sonic™ No. 2,** 1 21
Jr. Burger, 1 9

Toaster® Sandwiches

Bacon Cheddar Burger, 1 16
BLT, 1 14
Chicken Club, 1 15
Country Fried Steak, 1 17
Grilled Cheese, 1 6

Sandwiches

Country Fried Steak Sandwich, 1 18
Sonic® Bacon Egg & Cheese Toaster®, 1 12
Sonic® Ham Egg & Cheese Toaster®, 1 10
Sonic® Sausage Egg & Cheese Toaster®, 1 14

Chicken

Breaded Chicken Sandwich, 1 13
Chicken Strip Dinner, 1 serving 17
Grilled Chicken Sandwich, 1 8

Coneys

Regular Coney Plain, 1 6
Regular Cheese Coney, 1 9

POINTS

Extra Long Coney Plain, 1 12
Extra Long Cheese Coney, 1 16
Corn Dog, 1 6

Wraps

Chicken Strip Wrap, 1 14
Chicken Strip Wrap without Ranch, 1 9
Grilled Chicken Wrap, 1 13
Grilled Chicken Wrap without Ranch, 1 8

WackyPack® KidsMeal

Chicken Strips, 2 4
Corn Dog, 1 6
Hot Dog Plain, 1 6
Jr. Burger, 1 9
Regular French Fries, 1 serving 4
Regular Tater Tots, 1 serving 6

Faves&Craves™

Ched 'R' Peppers®, 1 serving 5
Cheese Fries, 1 regular serving 6
Cheese Fries, 1 large serving 8
Cheese Tater Tots, 1 regular serving 8
Cheese Tater Tots, 1 large serving 11
Chili Cheese Fries, 1 regular serving 7
Chili Cheese Fries, 1 large serving 8
Chili Cheese Tater Tots, 1 regular serving 9
Chili Cheese Tater Tots, 1 large serving 14
French Fries, 1 regular serving 4
French Fries, 1 large serving 5
French Fries, 1 Sonic-Size™ serving 8

POINTS

Fritos® Chili Pie, 1 serving 15
Mozzarella Sticks, 1 serving 9
Onion Rings, 1 regular serving 6
Onion Rings, 1 large serving 9
Onion Rings, 1 Sonic-Size™ serving 10
Tater Tots, 1 regular serving 6
Tater Tots, 1 large serving 9
Tater Tots, 1 Sonic-Size™ serving 12

FrozenFavorites® SonicBlast®

M&M®, 1 regular 15
M&M®, 1 large 20
Oreo®, 1 regular 15
Oreo®, 1 large 20
Reese's®, 1 regular 15
Reese's®, 1 large 21

FrozenFavorites® Floats

Blue Coconut Slush Float, 1 regular 9
Blue Coconut Slush Float, 1 large 14
Cherry Slush Float, 1 regular 9
Cherry Slush Float, 1 large 14
Coca-Cola® Float, 1 regular 9
Coca-Cola® Float, 1 large 12
Dr Pepper® Float, 1 regular 9
Dr Pepper® Float, 1 large 12
Grape Slush Float, 1 regular 9
Grape Slush Float, 1 large 14
Orange Slush Float, 1 regular 9
Orange Slush Float, 1 large 14
Rootbeer Float, 1 regular 9
Rootbeer Float, 1 large 12

POINTS

Watermelon Slush Float, 1 regular 10
Watermelon Slush Float, 1 large 14

FrozenFavorites® CreamSlush™Treats

Blue Coconut, 1 regular 9
Blue Coconut, 1 large 14
Cherry, 1 regular 9
Cherry, 1 large 14
Coca-Cola®, 1 regular 9
Coca-Cola®, 1 large 12
Dr Pepper®, 1 regular 9
Dr Pepper®, 1 large 12
Grape, 1 regular 9
Grape, 1 large 14
Orange, 1 regular 9
Orange, 1 large 14
Rootbeer, 1 regular 9
Rootbeer, 1 large 12
Watermelon, 1 regular 10
Watermelon, 1 large 14

Frozen Favorites® Premi-YUM™Shakes, Shakes&Malts

Banana Cream Pie Shake, 1 regular 17
Banana Cream Pie Shake, 1 large 23
Banana Shake, 1 regular 11
Banana Shake, 1 large 16
Chocolate Cream Pie Shake,
1 regular 18
Chocolate Cream Pie Shake, 1 large 25
Chocolate Shake, 1 regular 13
Chocolate Shake, 1 large 17

Frozen Favorites® Premi-YUM™ Shakes, Shakes & Malts (con't)

POINTS

Coconut Cream Pie Shake, 1 regular....16
Coconut Cream Pie Shake, 1 large........23
Pineapple Shake, 1 regular....................14
Pineapple Shake, 1 large.........................18
Strawberry Shake, 1 regular...................12
Strawberry Shake, 1 large.......................15
Vanilla Shake, 1 regular..........................11
Vanilla Shake, 1 large...............................14
Malt, 1 serving (may be added to any shake)..2

FrozenFavorites® SoftServe&Sundaes

Banana Split, 1..10
Chocolate Sundae, 1..................................8
Dish of Vanilla, 1 serving..........................6
Hot Fudge Sundae, 1..................................9
Pineapple Sundae, 1..................................9
Soft Serve Cone, 1.....................................7
Strawberry Sundae, 1..................................7

FountainFavorites® Drinks

Cherry Limeade, 1 regular.........................4
Cherry Limeade, 1 large.............................7
Limeade, 1 regular.......................................3
Limeade, 1 large...6
Ocean Water®, 1 regular............................4
Ocean Water®, 1 large.................................7
Strawberry Limeade, 1 regular...............4
Strawberry Limeade, 1 large...................6

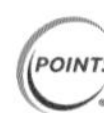

Breakfast

Breakfast Burrito, 1...............................18
Sonic French ToastSticks, 4...................10
Sonic Sunrise® Drink Regular, 1............4
Sonic Sunrise® Drink Large, 1................7

MealIdeas

2 Wacky Pack® Kids Meal Chicken Strips
1 serving Regular French Fries

1 Grilled Cheese Toaster® Sandwich
1 regular Ocean Water® Fountain Favorites® Drink

1 Jr. Burger
1 regular Limeade Fountain Favorites® Drink

Souplantation®

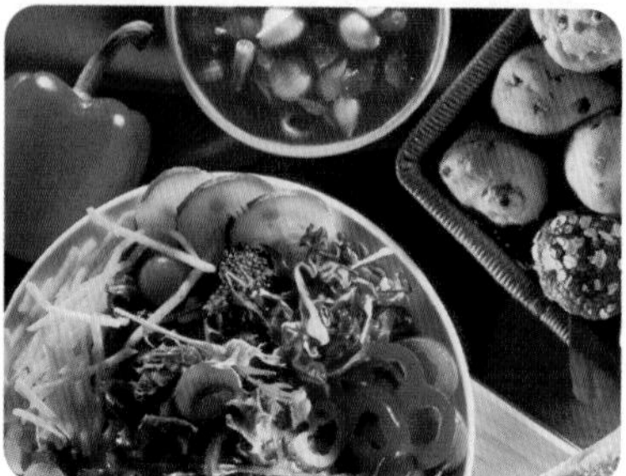

POINTS

FreshTossedSalads

Bartlett Pear & Walnut Salad, 1 cup.....4
BBQ Julienne Chopped Salad, 1 cup......4
Caesar Salad Asiago, 1 cup......................5
California Cobb Salad, 1 cup...................4
Cape Cod Spinach with Walnuts, 1 cup..4
Chicken Tortilla Salad, 1 cup...................4
Classic Antipasto Salad with Peppered Salami, 1 cup 3
Country Fresh Salad with Bacon, 1 cup..5
Ensalada Azteca Salad, 1 cup 3
Greek Salad, 1 cup....................................3
Italian Sub Salad with Turkey & Salami, 1 cup...6
Lox & Bagels Salad, 1 cup........................3
Mandarin Spinach Salad with Carmelized Walnuts, 1 cup 4
Mediterranean Salad, 1 cup 3
Monterey Blue Salad with Peanuts, 1 cup..5
Pesto Orzo Salad with Pinenuts, 1 cup..5

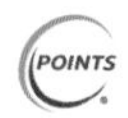

Ranch House BLT Salad with Turkey, 1 cup 4
Roasted Vegetables Salad with Feta & Olives, 1 cup 3
Roma Tomato, Mozzarella & Basil Salad, 1 cup...3
Smoked Turkey & Spinach Salad with Almonds, 1 cup 4
Sonoma Spinach Salad with Honey Dijon Vinaigrette, 1 cup 5
Spiced Pecan & Roasted Vegetable, 1 cup..4
Spinach Gorgonzola with Spiced Pecans, 1 cup 5
Strawberry Fields with Carmelized Walnuts, 1 cup 3
Summer Lemon with Spiced Pecans, 1 cup..5
Traditional Spinach Salad with Bacon, 1 cup 4
Watercress & Orange Salad, 1 cup 2
Won Ton Chicken Happiness, 1 cup 3

SignaturePreparedSalads

Ambrosia with Coconut, ½ cup 4
Artichoke Rice Salad, ½ cup....................3
Aunt Doris' Red Pepper Slaw (Fat-free), ½ cup 1
Baja Bean & Cilantro Salad (Low-fat), ½ cup...3
BBQ Potato Salad, ½ cup..........................3
Carrot Ginger Salad with Herb Vinaigrette, ½ cup....................................3
Carrot Raisin Salad (Low-fat), ½ cup....2
Chinese Krab Salad, ½ cup......................3

POINTS

Citrus Noodles Salad with Snow Peas, ½ cup....3
Dijon Potato Salad with Garlic Dill Vinaigrette, ½ cup....3
German Potato Salad (Low-fat), ½ cup....2
Greek Couscous Salad with Feta Cheese, ½ cup....4
Italian Garden Vegetable Salad, ½ cup....2
Italian White Bean Salad, ½ cup....2
Jalapeno Potato Salad, ½ cup....3
Joan's Broccoli Madness Salad, ½ cup....4
Lemon Rice with Cashews, ½ cup....4
Mandarin Noodles Salad with Broccoli (Low-fat), ½ cup....2
Mandarin Shells Salad with Almonds, ½ cup....2
Marinated Summer Vegetables Salad (Fat-free), ½ cup....1
Moroccan Marinated Vegetables Salad (Low-fat), ½ cup....2
Old Fashioned Macaroni Salad with Ham, ½ cup....4
Oriental Ginger Slaw with Krab (Low-fat), ½ cup....1
Penne Pasta Salad with Chicken in a Citrus Vinaigrette (Low-fat), ½ cup....2
Pesto Pasta Salad, ½ cup....3
Picnic Potato Salad, ½ cup....3
Pineapple Coconut Slaw, ½ cup....3
Poppyseed Coleslaw, ½ cup....3
Red Potato & Tomato, ½ cup....3
Roasted Potato Sald with Chipotle Chile Vinaigrette, ½ cup....3

POINTS

Shrimp & Seafood Shells Salad, ½ cup....5
Southern Dill Potato Salad (Low-fat), ½ cup....2
Southwestern Rice & Beans Salad, ½ cup....1
Spicy Southwestern Pasta Salad (Low-fat), ½ cup....2
Summer Barley Salad with Black Beans (Low-fat), ½ cup....2
Thai Noodle Salad with Peanut Sauce, ½ cup....3
Three Bean Marinated Salad, ½ cup....3
Tomato Cucumber Marinade Salad, ½ cup....2
Tuna Tarragon Salad, ½ cup....5
Turkey Chutney Pasta Salad, ½ cup....5
Wild Rice & Chicken Salad, ½ cup....8
Zesty Tortellini Salad, ½ cup....5

Salad Dressings & Croutons

Bacon Dressing, 2 Tbsp....3
Balsamic Vinaigrette, 2 Tbsp....5
Basil Vinaigrette, 2 Tbsp....5
Blue Cheese Dressing, 2 Tbsp....4
Creamy Italian Dressing, 2 Tbsp....3
Cucumber Dressing (Reduced Calorie), 2 Tbsp....2
Fat Free Honey Mustard Dressing (Fat-free), 2 Tbsp....1
Fat Free Italian Dressing (Fat-free), 2 Tbsp....0
Fat Free Ranch Dressing (Fat-free), 2 Tbsp....1
Garlic Parmesan Seasoned Croutons (Low-fat), 5 pieces....1

Salad Dressings & Croutons (con't) POINTS

Honey Mustard Dressing, 2 Tbsp 4
Kahlena French Dressing, 2 Tbsp............3
Parmesan Pepper Cream Dressing, 2 Tbsp............5
Ranch Dressing, 2 Tbsp............4
Roasted Garlic Dressing, 2 Tbsp 4
Thousand Island Dressing, 2 Tbsp 3
Tomato Basil Croutons, 5 pieces.............1

Soups&Chilies

Albondigas Buenas (A Meatball Soup), 1 cup............4
Arizona Chili, 1 cup............4
Baked Potato & Cheese with Bacon, 1 cup 7
Big Chunk Chicken Noodle (Low-fat), 1 cup 3
Butternut Squash Soup (Vegetarian), 1 cup............3
Chesapeake Corn Chowder, 1 cup 6
Chicken Fajitas & Black Bean Soup, 1 cup 5
Chicken Tortilla Soup with Jalapeno Chilies & Tomatoes (Low-fat), 1 cup....2
Chunky Potato Cheese Soup with Thyme, 1 cup 5
Country Corn & Red Potato Chowder, 1 cup 3
Cream of Broccoli Soup (Vegetarian), 1 cup............5
Cream of Chicken Soup, 1 cup............6
Cream of Mushroom Soup, 1 cup 7
Creamy Vegetable Chowder, 1 cup 4
Deep Kettle House Chili (Low-fat), 1 cup 5

POINTS

Deep Kettle Chili (with 33% more meat), 1 cup 5
El Paso Lime & Chicken Soup, 1 cup 3
French Onion Soup (Low-fat), 1 cup......2
Garden Fresh Vegetable Soup (Low-fat), 1 cup 1
Green Chile Stew, 1 cup 3
Hungarian Vegetable (Low-fat), 1 cup 2
Irish Potato Leek Soup (Vegetarian), 1 cup 6
Longhorn Beef Chili, 1 cup............4
Manhattan Clam Chowder, 1 cup...........3
Marvelous Minestrone Soup, 1 cup 4
Minestrone with Italian Sausage, 1 cup 4
Mulligatawny Soup, 1 cup 5
Navy Bean Soup with Ham, 1 cup 7
Old Fashioned Vegetable Soup (Low-fat/Vegetarian/No Cholesterol), 1 cup 1
Posole Soup, 1 cup............3
Santa Fe Black Bean Chili (Low-fat/ Vegetarian), 1 cup 3
Shrimp Bisque, 1 cup............7
Southwest Tomato Cream Soup, 1 cup 3
Spicy 4-Bean Minestrone (Low-fat/ Vegetarian), 1 cup 2
Spicy Sausage & Pasta Soup, 1 cup 6
Split Pea Soup with Ham, 1 cup 7
Sweet Tomato Cream Soup, 1 cup..........4
Sweet Tomato Onion Soup (Low-fat/ Vegetarian), 1 cup 2
Texas Red Chili, 1 cup 5

POINTS

Three-Bean Turkey Chili (Low-fat/ High Fiber/No Dairy), 1 cup 2
Tomato Parmesan & Vegetables (Low-fat/Vegetarian/with Dairy), 1 cup 2
Tortellini Soup, 1 cup 4
Turkey Vegetable Soup, 1 cup 6
Tuscany Chicken Stew, 1 cup 4
Vegetable Beef Stew, 1 cup 5
Vegetable Medley Soup (Low-fat/ Vegetarian), 1 cup 1
Vegetarian Chili (Vegetarian), 1 cup 2
Vegetarian Harvest Soup (Vegetarian), 1 cup 4
Vegetarian Lentils & Brown Rice (Low-fat/Vegetarian), 1 cup 2
Yankee Clipper Clam Chowder with Bacon, 1 cup 8

HotTossed**Pastas**

Broccoli Alfredo with Basil, 1 cup 9
Bruschetta, 1 cup 5
Carbonara Pasta, 1 cup 6
Cilantro Lime Pesto, 1 cup 9
Creamy Bruschetta, 1 cup 8
Creamy Herb Chicken, 1 cup 7
Creamy Pepper Jack, 1 cup 7
Fettuccine Alfredo, 1 cup 9
Garden Vegetable with Italian Sausage, 1 cup 6
Garden Vegetable with Meatballs, 1 cup 5
Greek Mediterranean, 1 cup 6
Italian Sausage with Red Pepper Puree, 1 cup 5

POINTS

Italian Vegetable Beef, 1 cup 5
Jalapeño Salsa, 1 cup 5
Lemon Cream & Asparagus, 1 cup 5
Linguini with Clam Sauce, 1 cup 8
Macaroni & Cheese, 1 cup 5
Nutty Mushroom, 1 cup 9
Oriental Green Bean & Noodle (Low-fat), 1 cup 5
Pasta Florentine, 1 cup 7
Smoked Salmon & Dill, 1 cup 8
Southwestern Alfredo Pasta, 1 cup 8
Tuscany Sausage with Capers & Olives, 1 cup 5
Vegetable Ragu, 1 cup 5
Vegetarian Marinara with Basil, 1 cup 5
Walnut Pesto, 1 cup 7

FreshBaked**Muffins**&**Breads**

Apple Cinnamon Bran Muffin (96% fat free), 1 1
Apple Raisin Muffin, 1 3
Banana Nut Muffin, 1 3
Big Blue Blueberry Muffin, 1 small 3
Big Blue Blueberry Muffin, 1 large 7
Big Hearth Focaccia (Low-fat), 1 2
Black Forest Muffin, 1 5
Bruschetta Focaccia, 1 3
Buttermilk Cornbread (Low-fat), 1 3
Cappuccino Chip Muffin, 1 3
Caribbean Key Lime Muffin, 1 4
Carrot Pineapple Muffin with Oat Bran, 1 3
Cherry Nut Muffin, 1 3

Fresh Baked Muffins & Breads (con't)

POINTS

Chile Corn Muffin (Low-fat), 1 3
Chocolate Brownie Muffin, 1 4
Chocolate Chip Muffin, 1 4
Country Blackberry Muffin, 1 4
Cranberry Orange Bran Muffin (96% Fat-free), 1 1
Fruit Medley Bran Muffin (96% Fat-free), 1 1
Garlic Parmesan Focaccia (Low-fat), 1 2
Georgia Peach Poppyseed Muffin, 1 3
Indian Grain Bread (Low-fat), 1 4
Lemon Muffin, 1 3
Macadamia Nut Spice Muffin, 1 5
Maple Walnut Muffin, 1 5
Nutty Peanut Butter Muffin, 1 4
Pauline's Apple Walnut Cake, 1 4
Pumpkin Raisin Muffin, 1 3
Roasted Potato Focaccia, 1 3
Sauteed Vegetable Focaccia, 1 3
Sourdough Bread (Low-fat), 1 3
Strawberry Buttermilk Muffin, 1 3
Sweet Orange & Cranberry Muffin, 1 4
Taffy Apple Muffin, 1 4
Tomatillo Focaccia, 1 3
Tropical Papaya Coconut Muffin, 1 4
Zucchini Nut Muffin, 1 3

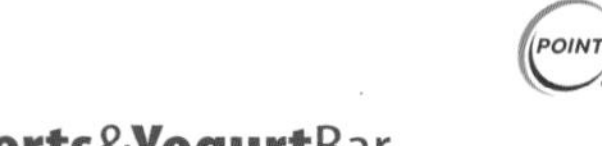

Desserts & Yogurt Bar Toppings

Apple Cobbler, ½ cup 8
Apple Medley (Fat-free), ½ cup 1
Banana Pudding, ½ cup 3
Banana Royale (Fat-free), ½ cup 1
Blissful Blueberry Cobbler, ½ cup 8
Butterscotch Pudding (Low-fat), ½ cup 3
Cherry Cobbler, ½ cup 7
Chocolate Chip Cookie, 1 small 2
Chocolate Lava Cake, ½ cup 7
Chocolate Pudding (Low-fat) (No Sugar Added), ½ cup 2
Chocolate Pudding (Low-fat), ½ cup 3
Cranberry Apple Cobbler, ½ cup 8
Ghirardelli Chocolate Frozen Yogurt (Fat-free), ½ cup 2
Jello (Flavored) (Fat-free), ½ cup 2
Jello (Sugar Free) (Flavored), ½ cup 0
Nutty Waldorf Salad (Low-fat), ½ cup 1
Rice Pudding (Low-fat), ½ cup 2
Tapioca Pudding (Low-fat), ½ cup 3
Vanilla Pudding, ½ cup 3
Vanilla Soft Serve (Reduced-fat), ½ cup 3
Candy Sprinkles (Low-fat), 1 Tbsp 2
Chocolate Syrup (Fat-free), 2 Tbsp 1
Granola Topping, 2 Tbsp 2

Meal Ideas

1 cup Old Fashioned Vegetable Soup
1 cup Classic Antipasto Salad with Peppered Salami
1 Cranberry Orange Bran Muffin
½ cup Banana Royale

1 cup Ensalada Azteca Salad
1 cup Arizona Chili
1 small Chocolate Chip Cookie

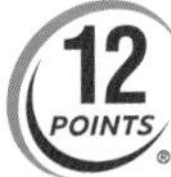

1 cup Carbonara Pasta
1 Bruschetta Focaccia
½ cup Vanilla Soft Serve

Starbucks Coffee®

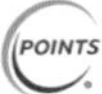

Beverages

Caffé Latte, made with nonfat milk, 1 tall (12 fl oz) 2

Caffé Latte, made with nonfat milk, 1 grande (16 fl oz) 3

Caffé Latte, made with whole milk, 1 tall (12 fl oz) 5

Caffé Mocha, made with nonfat milk and without whipped cream, 1 grande (16 fl oz) 4

Caffé Mocha, made with nonfat milk and whipped cream, 1 tall (12 fl oz) 6

Caffé Mocha, made with nonfat milk and whipped cream, 1 grande (16 fl oz) 8

Caffé Mocha, made with whole milk and without whipped cream, 1 tall (12 fl oz) 6

Cappuccino, made with nonfat milk, 1 tall (12 fl oz) 2

Cappuccino, made with whole milk, 1 tall (12 fl oz) 3

Coffee Frappuccino® blended coffee, 1 tall (12 fl oz) 4

Tazoberry® Frappuccino® blended tea, without whipped cream, 1 grande (16 fl oz) 4

Some Low-*POINT* Ideas

each

1 tall Caffé Latte (made with nonfat milk)

1 tall Cappuccino (made with nonfat milk)

each

1 grande Caffé Latte (made with nonfat milk)

1 tall Cappuccino (made with whole milk)

each

1 grande Caffé Mocha (made with nonfat milk, without whipped cream)

1 tall Coffee Frappuccino® blended coffee

1 grande Tazoberry® Frappuccino® blended tea (without whipped cream)

SUBWAY® Restaurants (United States)

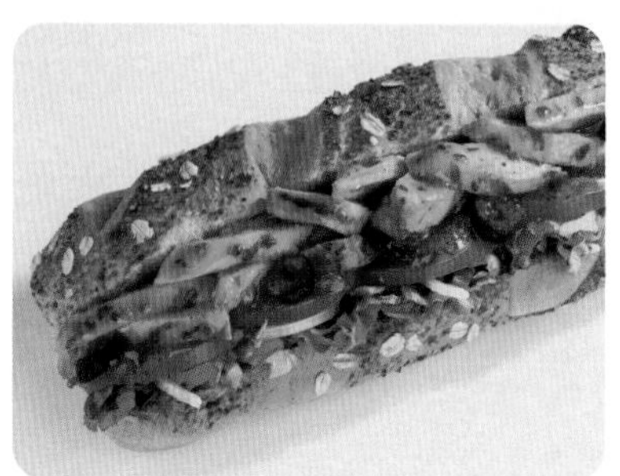

POINTS®

7 Sandwiches & Salads with 6 Grams of Fat or Less
(Low Fat)

7 Subs with 6 grams of fat or less (with standard vegetables)

Ham Sub, 6-inch 5
Roast Beef Sub, 6-inch 5
Roasted Chicken Breast Sub, 6-inch 6
Subway Club® Sub, 6-inch 6
Turkey Breast & Ham Sub, 6-inch 5
Turkey Breast Sub, 6-inch 5
Veggie Delite® Sub, 6-inch 4

Deli Style Sandwiches with 6 grams of fat or less (on deli style roll, with standard vegetables)

Ham Sandwich, 1 4
Roast Beef Sandwich, 1 4
Turkey Breast Sandwich, 1 4

7 Salads with 6 grams of fat or less (without cheese or salad dressing)

Ham Salad, 1 2

POINTS®

Roast Beef Salad, 1 2
Roasted Chicken Salad, 1 2
Subway Club® Salad, 1 3
Turkey Breast & Ham Salad, 1 2
Turkey Breast Salad, 1 2
Veggie Delite® Salad, 1 0

SUBWAY® Classics

Six-Inch SUBWAY® Classic Subs
(with standard vegetables, cheese and oil)

Cold Cut Trio™ Sub, 6-inch 10
Italian B.M.T.® Sub, 6-inch 11
Meatball Sub, 6-inch 12
Steak & Cheese Sub, 6-inch 8
Subway Melt® Sub, 6-inch 9
Subway Seafood & Crab® (a processed seafood & crab blend) Sub, made with light mayonnaise, 6-inch 9
Tuna Sub, made with light mayonnaise, 6-inch 10

SUBWAY® Classic Deli Style Sandwich (on deli style roll with standard vegetables, cheese and oil)

Tuna Sandwich, made with light mayonnaise, 1 7

SUBWAY® Classic Salads (with cheese, without salad dressing)

Cold Cut Trio™ Salad, 1 5
Italian B.M.T.® Salad, 1 7
Meatball Salad, 1 7
Steak & Cheese Salad, 1 3

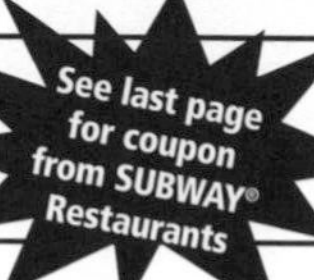

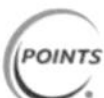

Subway Melt® Salad, 1 4
Subway Seafood & Crab® (a processed seafood & crab blend) Salad, made with light mayonnaise, 1 4
Tuna Salad, made with light mayonnaise, 1 6

Six-Inch SUBWAY® Select Subs
(with selected vegetables & select sauce)

Dijon Horseradish Melt, 6-inch 10
Honey Mustard Ham, 6-inch 6
Red Wine Vinaigrette Club, 6-inch 7
Southwest Turkey Bacon, 6-inch 9
Sweet Onion Chicken Teriyaki, 6-inch 7

Salad Dressings

Fat-Free French Dressing, 1 packet (4 Tbsp) 1
Fat-Free Italian Dressing, 1 packet (4 Tbsp) 0
Fat-Free Ranch Dressing, 1 packet (4 Tbsp) 1

Cookies

Chocolate Chip Cookie, 1 5
Chocolate Chunk Cookie, 1 5
Double Chocolate Chip, 1 5
M&M® Cookie, 1 5
Oatmeal Raisin Cookie, 1 4
Peanut Butter Cookie, 1 5
Sugar Cookie, 1 6
White Chocolate Macadamia Nut Cookie, 1 5

Meal Ideas

6-inch Low Fat Turkey Breast & Ham Sub (with standard vegetables)
1 Low Fat Veggie Delite® Salad (without cheese) with 1 packet Fat Free French Dressing

1 Low Fat Deli Style Roast Beef Sandwich (with standard vegetables)
1 Low Fat Veggie Delite® Salad (without cheese) with 1 packet Fat Free Italian Dressing
1 Oatmeal Raisin Cookie

6-inch SUBWAY® Select Southwest Turkey Bacon Sub
1 Low Fat Veggie Delite® Salad (without cheese) with 1 packet Fat Free Ranch Dressing

SUBWAY® Restaurants (Canada)

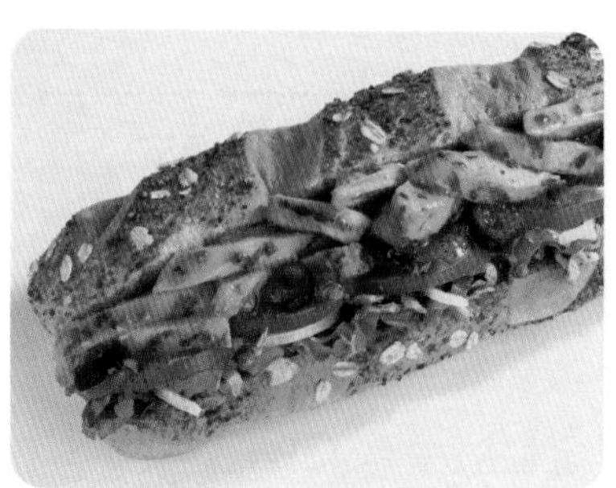

7 Sandwiches & Salads 6 Grams of Fat or Less

7 Subs with 6 grams of fat or less (with standard vegetables)

Ham Sub, 6-inch 5
Roast Beef Sub, 6-inch 5
Roasted Chicken Sub, 6-inch 6
Subway Club™ Sub, 6-inch 5
Turkey Breast & Ham Sub, 6-inch 5
Turkey Breast Sub, 6-inch 5
Veggie Delite™ Sub, 6-inch 4

Deli Style Sandwiches with 6 grams of fat or less (on deli style roll, with standard vegetables)

Ham Sandwich, 1 4
Roast Beef Sandwich, 1 4
Turkey Breast Sandwich, 1 4

7 Salads with 6 grams of fat or less (without cheese or salad dressing)

Ham Salad, 1 2
Roast Beef Salad, 1 2
Roasted Chicken Salad, 1 3
Subway Club™ Salad, 1 2
Turkey Breast & Ham Salad, 1 2
Turkey Breast Salad, 1 1
Veggie Delite™ Salad, 1 0

SUBWAY® Classics

Six-Inch SUBWAY® Classic Subs (with standard vegetables, cheese and oil)

Cold Cut Trio Sub, 6-inch 11
Italian B.M.T.® Sub, 6-inch 11
Meatball Sub, 6-inch 12
Steak & Cheese Sub, 6-inch 8
Subway Melt™ Sub, 6-inch 9
Subway Seafood & Crab™ (a processed seafood & crab blend) Sub, made with light mayonnaise-type dressing, 6-inch 9
Tuna Sub, made with light mayonnaise-type dressing, 6-inch 11

SUBWAY® Classic Deli Style Sandwich (on deli style roll, with standard vegetables, cheese and oil)

Tuna Sandwich, made with light mayonnaise-type dressing, 1 8

SUBWAY® Classic Salads (with cheese, without salad dressing)

Cold Cut Trio Salad, 1 7
Italian B.M.T.® Salad, 1 6
Meatball Salad, 1 8

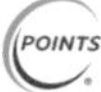

Steak & Cheese Salad, 1 3
Subway Melt™ Salad, 1 4
Subway Seafood & Crab™ (a processed seafood & crab blend) Salad, made with light mayonnaise-type dressing), 1 4
Tuna Salad, made with light mayonnaise-type dressing, 1 6

Six-inch SUBWAY® Select Subs

(with selected vegetables and select sauce)

Dijon Horseradish Melt, 6-inch 10
Honey Mustard Ham, 6-inch 6
Red Wine Vinaigrette Club, 6-inch 6
Southwest Turkey Bacon, 6-inch 8
Sweet Onion Chicken Teriyaki, 6-inch 7

Salad Dressings

Lite Italian Dressing, 2 Tbsp 1
Ranch Dressing, 2 Tbsp 5
Thousand Island Dressing, 2 Tbsp 3

Cookies

Chocolate chip, 1 5
Chocolate Chunk Cookie, 1 5
Double Chocolate Chip Cookie, 1 5
M&M® Cookie, 1 5
Oatmeal Raisin Cookie, 1 4
Peanut Butter Cookie, 1 5
Sugar, 1 6
White Chocolate Macadamia Nut Cookie, 1 5

Meal Ideas

6-inch Roast Beef Sub (with standard vegetables)
1 Turkey Breast Salad (without cheese) with 2 Tbsp Lite Italian Dressing

6-inch SUBWAY® Select Sweet Onion Chicken Teriyaki Sub (with selected vegetables and select sauce)
1 Veggie Delite™ Salad (without cheese) with 2 Tbsp Lite Italian Dressing

1 SUBWAY® Classic Deli Style Tuna Sandwich, made with light-type mayonnaise (with standard vegetables, cheese, and oil)
1 Veggie Delite™ Salad (without cheese) with 2 Tbsp Lite Italian Dressing

Sweet Tomatoes®

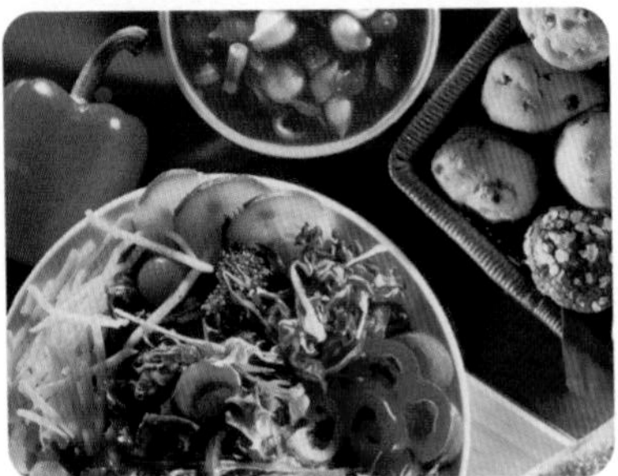

POINTS

Fresh Tossed Salads

Bartlett Pear & Walnut Salad, 1 cup 4
BBQ Julienne Chopped Salad, 1 cup 4
Caesar Salad Asiago, 1 cup 5
California Cobb Salad, 1 cup 4
Cape Cod Spinach with Walnuts, 1 cup 4
Chicken Tortilla Salad, 1 cup 4
Classic Antipasto Salad with Peppered Salami, 1 cup 3
Country Fresh Salad with Bacon, 1 cup 5
Ensalada Azteca Salad, 1 cup 3
Greek Salad, 1 cup 3
Italian Sub Salad with Turkey & Salami, 1 cup 6
Lox & Bagels Salad, 1 cup 3
Mandarin Spinach Salad with Carmelized Walnuts, 1 cup 4
Mediterranean Salad, 1 cup 3
Monterey Blue Salad with Peanuts, 1 cup 5
Pesto Orzo Salad with Pinenuts, 1 cup 5

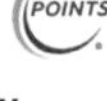

Ranch House BLT Salad with Turkey, 1 cup 4
Roasted Vegetables Salad with Feta & Olives, 1 cup 3
Roma Tomato, Mozzarella & Basil Salad, 1 cup 3
Smoked Turkey & Spinach Salad with Almonds, 1 cup 4
Sonoma Spinach Salad with Honey Dijon Vinaigrette, 1 cup 5
Spiced Pecan & Roasted Vegetable, 1 cup 4
Spinach Gorgonzola with Spiced Pecans, 1 cup 5
Strawberry Fields with Carmelized Walnuts, 1 cup 3
Summer Lemon with Spiced Pecans, 1 cup 5
Traditional Spinach Salad with Bacon, 1 cup 4
Watercress & Orange Salad, 1 cup 2
Won Ton Chicken Happiness, 1 cup 3

Signature Prepared Salads

Ambrosia with Coconut, ½ cup 4
Artichoke Rice Salad, ½ cup 3
Aunt Doris' Red Pepper Slaw (Fat-free), ½ cup 1
Baja Bean & Cilantro Salad (Low-fat), ½ cup 3
BBQ Potato Salad, ½ cup 3
Carrot Ginger Salad with Herb Vinaigrette, ½ cup 3
Carrot Raisin Salad (Low-fat), ½ cup 2
Chinese Krab Salad, ½ cup 3

POINTS

Citrus Noodles Salad with Snow Peas, ½ cup ... 3
Dijon Potato Salad with Garlic Dill Vinaigrette, ½ cup ... 3
German Potato Salad (Low-fat), ½ cup ... 2
Greek Couscous Salad with Feta Cheese, ½ cup ... 4
Italian Garden Vegetable Salad, ½ cup ... 2
Italian White Bean Salad, ½ cup ... 2
Jalapeno Potato Salad, ½ cup ... 3
Joan's Broccoli Madness Salad, ½ cup ... 4
Lemon Rice with Cashews, ½ cup ... 4
Mandarin Noodles Salad with Broccoli (Low-fat), ½ cup ... 2
Mandarin Shells Salad with Almonds, ½ cup ... 2
Marinated Summer Vegetables Salad (Fat-free), ½ cup ... 1
Moroccan Marinated Vegetables Salad (Low-fat), ½ cup ... 2
Old Fashioned Macaroni Salad with Ham, ½ cup ... 4
Oriental Ginger Slaw with Krab (Low-fat), ½ cup ... 1
Penne Pasta Salad with Chicken in a Citrus Vinaigrette (Low-fat), ½ cup ... 2
Pesto Pasta Salad, ½ cup ... 3
Picnic Potato Salad, ½ cup ... 3
Pineapple Coconut Slaw, ½ cup ... 3
Poppyseed Coleslaw, ½ cup ... 3
Red Potato & Tomato, ½ cup ... 3
Roasted Potato Sald with Chipotle Chile Vinaigrette, ½ cup ... 3

POINTS

Shrimp & Seafood Shells Salad, ½ cup ... 5
Southern Dill Potato Salad (Low-fat), ½ cup ... 2
Southwestern Rice & Beans Salad, ½ cup ... 1
Spicy Southwestern Pasta Salad (Low-fat), ½ cup ... 2
Summer Barley Salad with Black Beans (Low-fat), ½ cup ... 2
Thai Noodle Salad with Peanut Sauce, ½ cup ... 3
Three Bean Marinated Salad, ½ cup ... 3
Tomato Cucumber Marinade Salad, ½ cup ... 2
Tuna Tarragon Salad, ½ cup ... 5
Turkey Chutney Pasta Salad, ½ cup ... 5
Wild Rice & Chicken Salad, ½ cup ... 8
Zesty Tortellini Salad, ½ cup ... 5

Salad Dressings & Croutons

Bacon Dressing, 2 Tbsp ... 3
Balsamic Vinaigrette, 2 Tbsp ... 5
Basil Vinaigrette, 2 Tbsp ... 5
Blue Cheese Dressing, 2 Tbsp ... 4
Creamy Italian Dressing, 2 Tbsp ... 3
Cucumber Dressing (Reduced Calorie), 2 Tbsp ... 2
Fat Free Honey Mustard Dressing (Fat-free), 2 Tbsp ... 1
Fat Free Italian Dressing (Fat-free), 2 Tbsp ... 0
Fat Free Ranch Dressing (Fat-free), 2 Tbsp ... 1
Garlic Parmesan Seasoned Croutons (Low-fat), 5 pieces ... 1

Salad Dressings & Croutons (con't) POINTS

Honey Mustard Dressing, 2 Tbsp 4
Kahlena French Dressing, 2 Tbsp 3
Parmesan Pepper Cream Dressing, 2 Tbsp 5
Ranch Dressing, 2 Tbsp 4
Roasted Garlic Dressing, 2 Tbsp 4
Thousand Island Dressing, 2 Tbsp 3
Tomato Basil Croutons, 5 pieces 1

Soups&Chilies

Albondigas Buenas (A Meatball Soup), 1 cup 4
Arizona Chili, 1 cup 4
Baked Potato & Cheese with Bacon, 1 cup 7
Big Chunk Chicken Noodle (Low-fat), 1 cup 3
Butternut Squash Soup (Vegetarian), 1 cup 3
Chesapeake Corn Chowder, 1 cup 6
Chicken Fajitas & Black Bean Soup, 1 cup 5
Chicken Tortilla Soup with Jalapeno Chilies & Tomatoes (Low-fat), 1 cup 2
Chunky Potato Cheese Soup with Thyme, 1 cup 5
Country Corn & Red Potato Chowder, 1 cup 3
Cream of Broccoli Soup (Vegetarian), 1 cup 5
Cream of Chicken Soup, 1 cup 6
Cream of Mushroom Soup, 1 cup 7
Creamy Vegetable Chowder, 1 cup 4
Deep Kettle House Chili (Low-fat), 1 cup 5

POINTS

Deep Kettle Chili (with 33% more meat), 1 cup 5
El Paso Lime & Chicken Soup, 1 cup 3
French Onion Soup (Low-fat), 1 cup 2
Garden Fresh Vegetable Soup (Low-fat), 1 cup 1
Green Chile Stew, 1 cup 3
Hungarian Vegetable (Low-fat), 1 cup 2
Irish Potato Leek Soup (Vegetarian), 1 cup 6
Longhorn Beef Chili, 1 cup 4
Manhattan Clam Chowder, 1 cup 3
Marvelous Minestrone Soup, 1 cup 4
Minestrone with Italian Sausage, 1 cup 4
Mulligatawny Soup, 1 cup 5
Navy Bean Soup with Ham, 1 cup 7
Old Fashioned Vegetable Soup (Low-fat/Vegetarian/No Cholesterol), 1 cup 1
Posole Soup, 1 cup 3
Santa Fe Black Bean Chili (Low-fat/ Vegetarian), 1 cup 3
Shrimp Bisque, 1 cup 7
Southwest Tomato Cream Soup, 1 cup 3
Spicy 4-Bean Minestrone (Low-fat/ Vegetarian), 1 cup 2
Spicy Sausage & Pasta Soup, 1 cup 6
Split Pea Soup with Ham, 1 cup 7
Sweet Tomato Cream Soup, 1 cup 4
Sweet Tomato Onion Soup (Low-fat/ Vegetarian), 1 cup 2
Texas Red Chili, 1 cup 5

POINTS

Three-Bean Turkey Chili (Low-fat/ High Fiber/No Dairy), 1 cup 2
Tomato Parmesan & Vegetables (Low-fat/Vegetarian/with Dairy), 1 cup 2
Tortellini Soup, 1 cup 4
Turkey Vegetable Soup, 1 cup 6
Tuscany Chicken Stew, 1 cup 4
Vegetable Beef Stew, 1 cup 5
Vegetable Medley Soup (Low-fat/ Vegetarian), 1 cup 1
Vegetarian Chili (Vegetarian), 1 cup 2
Vegetarian Harvest Soup (Vegetarian), 1 cup 4
Vegetarian Lentils & Brown Rice (Low-fat/Vegetarian), 1 cup 2
Yankee Clipper Clam Chowder with Bacon, 1 cup 8

HotTossedPastas

Broccoli Alfredo with Basil, 1 cup 9
Bruschetta, 1 cup 5
Carbonara Pasta, 1 cup 6
Cilantro Lime Pesto, 1 cup 9
Creamy Bruschetta, 1 cup 8
Creamy Herb Chicken, 1 cup 7
Creamy Pepper Jack, 1 cup 7
Fettuccine Alfredo, 1 cup 9
Garden Vegetable with Italian Sausage, 1 cup 6
Garden Vegetable with Meatballs, 1 cup 5
Greek Mediterranean, 1 cup 6
Italian Sausage with Red Pepper Puree, 1 cup 5

POINTS

Italian Vegetable Beef, 1 cup 5
Jalapeño Salsa, 1 cup 5
Lemon Cream & Asparagus, 1 cup 5
Linguini with Clam Sauce, 1 cup 8
Macaroni & Cheese, 1 cup 5
Nutty Mushroom, 1 cup 9
Oriental Green Bean & Noodle (Low-fat), 1 cup 5
Pasta Florentine, 1 cup 7
Smoked Salmon & Dill, 1 cup 8
Southwestern Alfredo Pasta, 1 cup 8
Tuscany Sausage with Capers & Olives, 1 cup 5
Vegetable Ragu, 1 cup 5
Vegetarian Marinara with Basil, 1 cup 5
Walnut Pesto, 1 cup 7

FreshBakedMuffins&Breads

Apple Cinnamon Bran Muffin (96% fat free), 1 1
Apple Raisin Muffin, 1 3
Banana Nut Muffin, 1 3
Big Blue Blueberry Muffin, 1 small 3
Big Blue Blueberry Muffin, 1 large 7
Big Hearth Focaccia (Low-fat), 1 2
Black Forest Muffin, 1 5
Bruschetta Focaccia, 1 3
Buttermilk Cornbread (Low-fat), 1 3
Cappuccino Chip Muffin, 1 3
Caribbean Key Lime Muffin, 1 4
Carrot Pineapple Muffin with Oat Bran, 1 3
Cherry Nut Muffin, 1 3

Fresh Baked Muffins & Breads (con't) — POINTS

Chile Corn Muffin (Low-fat), 1 3
Chocolate Brownie Muffin, 1 4
Chocolate Chip Muffin, 1 4
Country Blackberry Muffin, 1 4
Cranberry Orange Bran Muffin (96% Fat-free), 1 1
Fruit Medley Bran Muffin (96% Fat-free), 1 1
Garlic Parmesan Focaccia (Low-fat), 1 2
Georgia Peach Poppyseed Muffin, 1 3
Indian Grain Bread (Low-fat), 1 4
Lemon Muffin, 1 3
Macadamia Nut Spice Muffin, 1 5
Maple Walnut Muffin, 1 5
Nutty Peanut Butter Muffin, 1 4
Pauline's Apple Walnut Cake, 1 4
Pumpkin Raisin Muffin, 1 3
Roasted Potato Focaccia, 1 3
Sauteed Vegetable Focaccia, 1 3
Sourdough Bread (Low-fat), 1 3
Strawberry Buttermilk Muffin, 1 3
Sweet Orange & Cranberry Muffin, 1 4
Taffy Apple Muffin, 1 4
Tomatillo Focaccia, 1 3
Tropical Papaya Coconut Muffin, 1 4
Zucchini Nut Muffin, 1 3

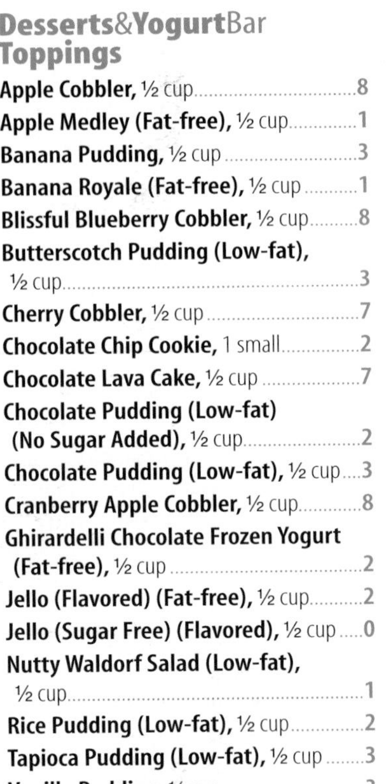

POINTS

Desserts & Yogurt Bar Toppings

Apple Cobbler, ½ cup 8
Apple Medley (Fat-free), ½ cup 1
Banana Pudding, ½ cup 3
Banana Royale (Fat-free), ½ cup 1
Blissful Blueberry Cobbler, ½ cup 8
Butterscotch Pudding (Low-fat), ½ cup 3
Cherry Cobbler, ½ cup 7
Chocolate Chip Cookie, 1 small 2
Chocolate Lava Cake, ½ cup 7
Chocolate Pudding (Low-fat) (No Sugar Added), ½ cup 2
Chocolate Pudding (Low-fat), ½ cup 3
Cranberry Apple Cobbler, ½ cup 8
Ghirardelli Chocolate Frozen Yogurt (Fat-free), ½ cup 2
Jello (Flavored) (Fat-free), ½ cup 2
Jello (Sugar Free) (Flavored), ½ cup 0
Nutty Waldorf Salad (Low-fat), ½ cup 1
Rice Pudding (Low-fat), ½ cup 2
Tapioca Pudding (Low-fat), ½ cup 3
Vanilla Pudding, ½ cup 3
Vanilla Soft Serve (Reduced-fat), ½ cup 3
Candy Sprinkles (Low-fat), 1 Tbsp 2
Chocolate Syrup (Fat-free), 2 Tbsp 1
Granola Topping, 2 Tbsp 2

MealIdeas

1 cup Old Fashioned Vegetable Soup
1 cup Classic Antipasto Salad with Peppered Salami
1 Cranberry Orange Bran Muffin
½ cup Banana Royale

1 cup Ensalada Azteca Salad
1 cup Arizona Chili
1 small Chocolate Chip Cookie

1 cup Carbonara Pasta
1 Bruschetta Focaccia
½ cup Vanilla Soft Serve

Taco Bell®

POINTS

Tacos

Taco (beef), 1 4
Taco Supreme® (beef), 1 5
Soft Taco (beef), 1 5
Soft Taco (chicken), 1 4
Soft Taco Supreme® (beef), 1 6
Soft Taco Supreme® (chicken), 1 5
Grilled Steak Soft Taco, 1 7
DOUBLE DECKER® Taco Supreme®, 1 8
DOUBLE DECKER® Taco, 1 7

Gorditas

Gordita Baja® (beef), 1 8
Gordita Baja® (chicken), 1 7
Gordita Baja® (steak), 1 7
Gordita Nacho Cheese (beef), 1 6
Gordita Nacho Cheese (chicken), 1 6
Gordita Nacho Cheese (steak), 1 6
Gordita Supreme® (beef), 1 7
Gordita Supreme® (chicken), 1 6
Gordita Supreme® (steak), 1 6

Chalupas

Chalupa Baja (beef), 1 10
Chalupa Baja (chicken), 1 10
Chalupa Baja (steak), 1 10
Chalupa Nacho Cheese (beef), 1 9
Chalupa Nacho Cheese (chicken), 1 8
Chalupa Nacho Cheese (steak), 1 8
Chalupa Supreme (beef), 1 9
Chalupa Supreme (chicken), 1 9
Chalupa Supreme (steak), 1 9

POINTS

Burritos

Bean Burrito, 1 7
Chili Cheese Burrito, 1 9
7-Layer Burrito, 1 12
Burrito Supreme® (beef), 1 10
Burrito Supreme® (chicken), 1 9
Burrito Supreme® (steak), 1 9
Fiesta Burrito (beef), 1 8
Fiesta Burrito (chicken), 1 8
Fiesta Burrito (steak), 1 8
Grilled Stuft Burrito (beef), 1 17
Grilled Stuft Burrito (chicken), 1 15
Grilled Stuft Burrito (steak), 1 15

Specialties

Cheese Quesadilla, 1 12
Chicken Quesadilla, 1 13
Enchirito® (beef), 1 8
Enchirito® (chicken), 1 7
Enchirito® (steak), 1 8
Express Taco Salad with Chips, 1 14
Extreme Cheese Quesadilla, 1 11
Mexican Pizza, 1 13
MexiMelt®, 1 7
Southwest Steak Bowl, 1 16
Steak Quesadilla, 1 13
Taco Salad, with salsa, without shell, 1 9
Taco Salad, with shell and salsa, 1 19
Tostada, 1 5
Zesty Chicken BORDER BOWL™, 1 17
Zesty Chicken BORDER BOWL™, without dressing, 1 11

Nachos&Sides

Nachos, 1 serving 8
Nachos Supreme, 1 serving 10
Nachos BellGrande®, 1 18
Mexican Rice, 1 serving 4
Pintos 'N Cheese, 1 serving 3
Cinnamon Twists, 1 serving 4

BreakfastItems

Breakfast Burrito, 1 11
Breakfast Gordita, 1 9
Breakfast Quesadilla, 1 9
Breakfast Steak Burrito, 1 12
Breakfast Steak Quesadilla with Green Sauce, 1 11

MealIdeas

1 Soft Taco (chicken)
1 serving Pintos 'N Cheese

1 Taco (beef)
1 serving Mexican Rice

1 Gordita Baja™ (steak)
1 serving Pintos 'N Cheese

TACO JOHN'S®

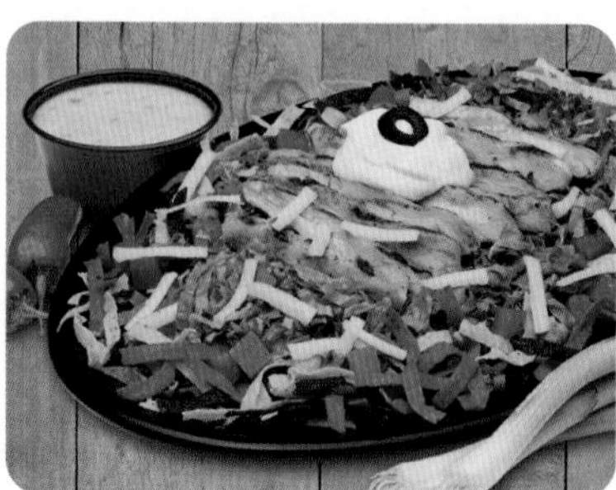

POINTS®

Tacos

Crispy Taco, 1 5
Sierra Taco™ - Beef, 1 12
Sierra Taco™ - Chicken, 1 11
Softshell Chicken Taco, 1 4
Softshell Taco, 1 5
Taco Bravo®, 1 8
Taco Burger, 1 6

Burritos

Bean Burrito, 1 8
Beefy Burrito, 1 10
Chicken & Potato Burrito, 1 10
Combination Burrito, 1 9
Meat & Potato Burrito, 1 11
Super Burrito, 1 10

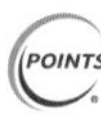

Specialties

Cheese Quesadilla, 1 11
Chicken Festiva Burrito, 1 13
Chicken Festiva Salad, with dressing, 1 18
Chicken Festiva Salad, without dressing, 1 9
Chicken Quesadilla, 1 12
Chicken Super Nachos, 1 serving 21
Potato Olés® Bravo, 1 serving 14
Super Nachos, 1 serving 22
Super Potato Olés®, 1 serving 24
Taco Salad, with dressing, 1 19
Taco Salad, without dressing, 1 14

Sides

Mexican Rice, 1 serving 5
Nachos, 1 serving 11
Potato Olés®, 1 kid's meal serving 7
Potato Olés®, 1 small serving 10
Potato Olés®, 1 medium serving 14
Potato Olés®, 1 large serving 18
Refried Beans, 1 serving 7
Side Salad, 1 serving 7
Texas Style Chili, 1 serving 7

Desserts

Apple Grande, 1 serving 6
Choco Taco, 1 7
Churros, 1 serving 4
Taco John's Cinnamon Mint Swirl, 1 0
Taco John's Cookies (Kid's Meal), 1 bag 3

LocalFavorites (not available at all locations)

Bean Tostada, 1 3
Beef & Bean Chimi Platter, 1 17
Beef Enchilada Platter, 1 18
Cheese Crisp, 1 6
Chicken Enchilada Platter, 1 16
Chicken Fajita Burrito, 1 7
Chilito, 1 10
Double Enchilada, 1 serving 18
El Grande Burrito, 1 17
El Grande Chicken Burrito, 1 15
El Grande Chicken Taco, 1 8
Mexi Rolls®, 1 serving 11
Potato Olés® with Nacho Cheese, 1 serving 13
Ranch Burrito - Beef, 1 10
Ranch Burrito - Chicken, 1 9
Smothered Burrito, 1 11
Smothered Burrito Platter, 1 19
Taco John's® Mexican Pizza, 1 13
Tostada, 1 5

MealIdeas

2 Softshell Chicken Tacos
1 Taco John's Cinnamon Mint Swirl

1 Softshell Taco
1 serving Mexican Rice

1 Crispy Taco
1 serving Apple Grande

TacoTime®

POINTS

Burritos

Beef, Bean & Cheese Burrito, 1 13
Big Juan® Burrito, 1 14
Casita Burrito®, made with meat, 1 ... 15
Chicken Big Juan® Burrito, 1 14
Chicken B.L.T. Burrito, 1 14
Chicken & Black Bean Burrito, 1 9
Crisp Bean Burrito, 1 9
Crisp Chicken Burrito, 1 10
Crisp Meat Burrito, 1 13
Soft Bean Burrito, 1 8
Soft Meat Burrito, 1 11
Veggie Burrito, 1 10

Tacos&Quesadilla

Cheddar Melt, 1 serving 5
Chicken Soft Taco, 1 8
Crisp Taco, 1 7
Soft Taco, 1 7
Super Soft Taco, 1 11
½ lb. Soft Flour Taco, 1 11
Taco Cheeseburger, 1 15

Salads

Chicken Taco Salad, without dressing, 1 regular serving 9
Taco Salad, without dressing, 1 regular serving 11
Tostada Salad, 1 15

Sides&Nachos

Cheddar Fries, 1 small serving 9
Cheddar Fries, 1 medium serving 13
Cheddar Fries, 1 large serving 18

POINTS

Mexi Fries®, 1 small serving 7
Mexi Fries®, 1 large serving 13
Mexi-Rice, 1 serving 3
Nachos, 1 serving 16
Nachos Deluxe, 1 serving 25
Refritos (with cheese and enchilada sauce), 1 serving 7
Stuffed Fries, 1 small serving 12
Stuffed Fries, 1 medium serving 16
Stuffed Fries, 1 large serving 25

Desserts

Cinnamon Crustos®, 1 serving 9
Empanada (cherry), 1 6

Condiments

Green Sauce, 1 serving (1 oz) 0
Guacamole, 1 serving (1 oz) 0
Original Hot Sauce, 1 serving (1 oz) 0
Ranch Dressing, 1 serving (1.5 oz) 4
Salsa Fresca, 1 serving (1 oz) 1
Sour Cream, 1 serving (1 oz) 2
1000 Island Dressing, 1 serving (1 oz) 5

Note: This information pertains only to the TacoTime® restaurants in the following areas: Oregon, Eastern and Southern Washington, Idaho, Utah, Montana, Colorado, Wyoming, Nevada, California, North Dakota, Iowa, Alaska and Connecticut.

MealIdeas

1 serving Cheddar Melt Quesadilla
1 serving Mexi-Rice

1 Soft Taco
1 serving Mexi-Rice

1 serving Cheddar Melt Quesadilla
1 serving Refritos (with cheese and enchilada sauce)

TCBY®

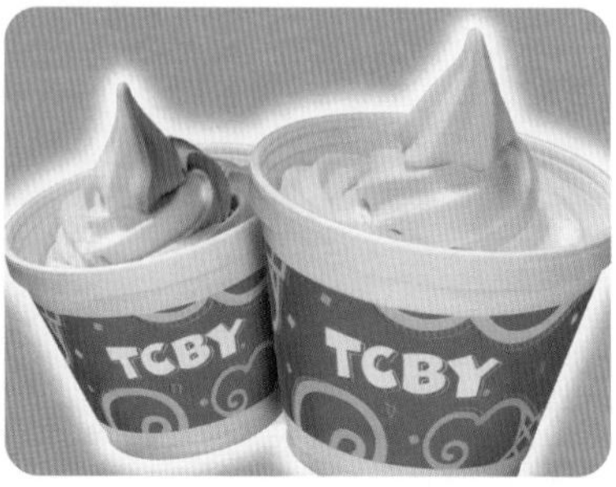

Regular Soft-Serve Frozen Yogurt (96% Fat Free)

Kiddie Cup, 1 serving 2
Junior Cup, 1 serving 4
Small Cup, 1 serving 5
Regular Cup, 1 serving 6
Large Cup, 1 serving 8

Nonfat Soft-Serve Frozen Yogurt

Kiddie Cup, 1 serving 2
Junior Cup, 1 serving 3
Small Cup, 1 serving 5
Regular Cup, 1 serving 6
Large Cup, 1 serving 7

Nonfat No-Sugar-Added Soft-Serve Frozen Yogurt

Kiddie Cup, 1 serving 1
Junior Cup, 1 serving 2
Small Cup, 1 serving 3
Regular Cup, 1 serving 4
Large Cup, 1 serving 4

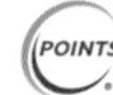

Sorbet

Kiddie Cup, 1 serving 1
Junior Cup, 1 serving 3
Small Cup, 1 serving 4
Regular Cup, 1 serving 5
Large Cup, 1 serving 6

Smoothie

Banana Berry Blast-Off, 1 regular serving 8
Latté Cooler, 1 regular serving 9
Mighty Berry, 1 regular serving 6
Passion Power, 1 regular serving 6
Peanut Butter Fusion, 1 regular serving 17
Piña Chill-Ada, 1 regular serving 9
Pineapple Combustion, 1 regular serving 7
Raging Raspberry, 1 regular serving 6
Raspberry Rush, 1 regular serving 7
Strawberry Surge, 1 regular serving 8
Tropical Bliss, 1 regular serving 7

Ice cream novelties*

Chocolate Sorbet, 1 bar 1
Orange Sorbet Swirl, 1 bar 2
Raspberry Sorbet Swirl, 1 bar 2

*May not be available at all locations.

Some Low-*POINT* Ideas

each

1 kiddie cup of Nonfat No-Sugar-Added Soft-Serve Frozen Yogurt
1 bar Chocolate Sorbet
1 kiddie cup of Sorbet

each

1 kiddie cup of Regular Soft-Serve Frozen Yogurt
1 kiddie cup of Nonfat Soft-Serve Frozen Yogurt
1 junior cup of Nonfat No-Sugar-Added Soft-Serve Frozen Yogurt
1 bar Orange or Raspberry Sorbet Swirl

each

1 junior cup of Nonfat Soft-Serve Frozen Yogurt
1 small cup of Nonfat No-Sugar-Added Soft-Serve Frozen Yogurt
1 junior cup of Sorbet

Tim Hortons® (United States)

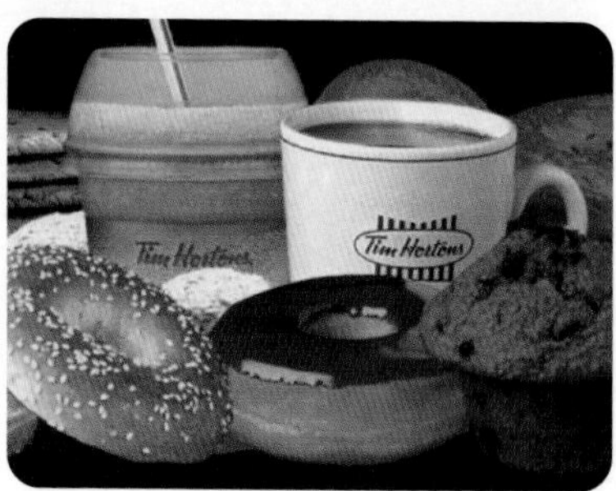

POINTS

Yeast Donuts

Apple Fritter Donut, 1 7
Chocolate Dip Donut, 1 5
Dutchie Donut, 1 6
Honey Dip Donut, 1 5
Maple Dip Donut, 1 6

Cake Donuts

Chocolate Glazed Donut, 1 9
Old Fashion Glazed Donut, 1 6
Old Fashion Plain Donut, 1 5
Sour Cream Plain Donut, 1 7

Filled Donuts

Angel Cream Donut, 1 7
Blueberry Filled Donut, 1 5
Boston Cream Donut, 1 5
Canadian Maple Donut, 1 5
Strawberry Filled Donut, 1 5

POINTS

Other Donuts

Honey Stick, 1 7
Sugar Twist, 1 5
Walnut Crunch Donut, 1 8

Yeast Timbits®

Dutchie Timbit, 1 1
Honey Dip Timbit, 1 1

Cake Timbits®

Chocolate Glazed Timbits, 1 2
Old Fashion Plain Timbit, 1 1

Filled Timbits®

Banana Cream Timbit, 1 1
Lemon Timbit, 1 1
Spiced Apple Timbit, 1 1
Strawberry Filled Timbit, 1 1

Muffins

Blueberry Bran Muffin, 1 6
Carrot Whole Wheat Muffin, 1 9
Chocolate Chip Plain Muffin, 1 9
Low Fat Carrot Muffin, 1 5
Low Fat Cranberry Muffin, 1 5
Low Fat Honey Muffin, 1 5
Oat Bran Carrot 'n Raisin Muffin, 1 7
Oat Bran 'n Apple Muffin, 1 7
Oatmeal Raisin Muffin, 1 9
Raisin Bran Muffin, 1 7
Wild Blueberry Muffin, 1 7

POINTS

Bagels (without spread)

Blueberry Bagel, 1 ... 6
Cinnamon Raisin Bagel, 1 ... 5
Everything Bagel, 1 ... 6
Multigrain Bagel, 1 ... 5
Onion Bagel, 1 ... 5
Plain Bagel, 1 ... 5
Poppy Seed Bagel, 1 ... 5
Sesame Seed Bagel, 1 ... 5
Whole Wheat & Honey Bagel, 1 ... 5

Cream Cheese

Garden Vegetable Cream Cheese, 3 Tbsp ... 4
Plain Cream Cheese, 3 Tbsp ... 4
Plain Light Cream Cheese, 3 Tbsp ... 2
Strawberry Cream Cheese, 3 Tbsp ... 4

Tim's Own™ Sandwiches

(on white bun)

Albacore Tuna Salad Sandwich, 1 ... 7
Black Forest Ham & Swiss Sandwich, 1 ... 15
Chunky Chicken Salad Sandwich, 1 ... 8
Fireside Roast Beef Sandwich, 1 ... 11
Garden Vegetable Sandwich, 1 ... 11
Harvest Turkey Breast Sandwich, 1 ... 11

POINTS

Soup & Chili

Chili, 1 bowl ... 6
Cream of Broccoli Soup, 1 bowl ... 4
Cream of Mushroom Soup, 1 bowl ... 5
Hearty Vegetable Soup, 1 bowl ... 2
Minestrone Soup, 1 bowl ... 2
Potato Bacon Soup, 1 bowl ... 4
Tim's Own™ Chicken Noodle Soup, 1 bowl ... 2
Turkey & Wild Rice Soup, 1 bowl ... 2
Vegetable Beef Barley Soup, 1 bowl ... 2

Pies

Apple Pie, 1 slice (¼ pie) ... 13
Banana Cream Pie, 1 slice (¼ pie) ... 11
Cherry Pie, 1 slice (¼ pie) ... 14
Chocolate Cream Pie, 1 slice (¼ pie) ... 12

Cakes

Black Forest Cake, with whipped cream, 1 slice ... 11
Celebration Cake (white), 1 slice (⅛ cake) ... 11
Chocolate Fantasy Cake, with whipped cream, 1 slice ... 9
Shadow Cake (white and chocolate), 1 slice (⅛ cake) ... 10

Tarts

Fresh Strawberry Tart, 1 ... 5
Raisin Butter Tart, 1 ... 7

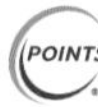

Baked Goods

Butter Croissant, 1 5
Cheese Croissant, 1 6
Cherry Cheese Danish, 1 9
Plain Tea Biscuits, 1 5
Raisin Tea Biscuit, 1 5
Southern Country Cranberry Biscuit, 1 11
Southern Country Raspberry Biscuit, 1 11

Cookies

Chocolate Chip Cookie, 1 3
Oatcake, 1 4
Oatmeal Raisin Cookie, 1 3
Peanut Butter Chocolate Chunk Cookie, 1 4
Peanut Butter Cookie, 1 4
Plain Macaroon, 1 3

Beverages

Café Mocha, 10 oz 6
Cappuccino ice, 16 oz 11
English Toffee Cappuccino, 10 oz 3
French Vanilla Cappuccino, 10 oz 3
Hot Chocolate, 10 oz 5

Meal Ideas

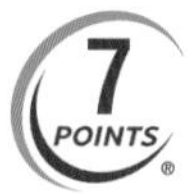

1 bowl Vegetable Beef Barley Soup
1 Low Fat Carrot Muffin

1 Old Fashion Plain Cake Donut
10 oz serving English Toffee Cappuccino

1 Tim's Own™ Albacore Tuna Salad Sandwich (on white bun)
1 bowl Hearty Vegetable Soup

Tim Hortons® (Canada)

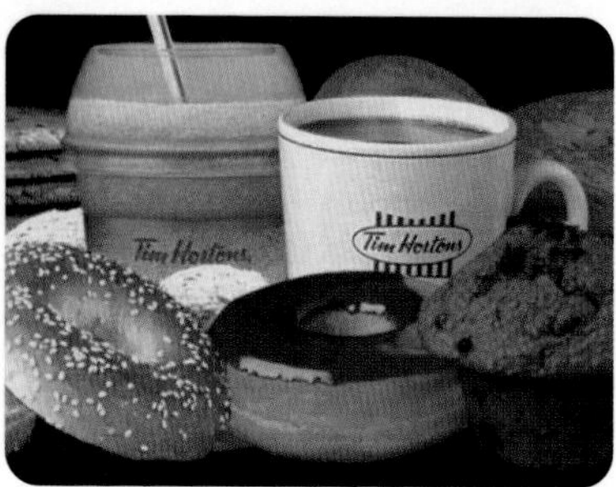

POINTS

YeastDonuts

Apple Fritter Donut, 1 8
Blueberry Fritter, 1 8
Chocolate Dip Donut, 1 5
Dutchie Donut, 1 7
Honey Dip Donut, 1 5
Maple Dip Donut, 1 6

CakeDonuts

Chocolate Glazed Donut, 1 9
Old Fashion Glazed Donut, 1 6
Old Fashion Plain Donut, 1 5
Sour Cream Glazed Donut, 1 8
Sour Cream Plain Donut, 1 7

FilledDonuts

Apple Dumpling Donut, 1 6
Blueberry Filled Donut, 1 6
Boston Cream Donut, 1 6
Canadian Maple Donut, 1 6
Strawberry Filled Donut, 1 6

POINTS

OtherDonuts

Honey Stick, 1 8
Sugar Twist, 1 5
Walnut Crunch Donut, 1 8

YeastTimbits®

Dutchie Timbit, 1 1
Honey Dip Timbit, 1 1

CakeTimbits®

Chocolate Glazed Timbit, 1 1
Old Fashion Plain Timbit, 1 1
Sour Cream Glazed Timbit, 1 1

FilledTimbits®

Banana Cream Timbit, 1 1
Lemon Timbit, 1 1
Spiced Apple Timbit, 1 1
Strawberry Filled Timbit, 1 1

Muffins

Blueberry Bran Muffin, 1 6
Blueberry Muffin, 1 7
Carrot Whole Wheat Muffin, 1 9
Chocolate Chip Plain Muffin, 1 9
Fruit Explosion, 1 7
Low Fat Carrot Muffin, 1 5
Low Fat Cranberry Muffin, 1 5
Low Fat Honey Muffin, 1 5
Oat Bran Carrot 'n Raisin Muffin, 1 7
Oat Bran 'n Apple Muffin, 1 7
Oatmeal Raisin Muffin, 1 9
Raisin Bran Muffin, 1 7

POINTS

Bagels (without spread)

Blueberry Bagel, 1 6
Chocolate Chunk Bagel, 1 6
Cinnamon Raisin Bagel, 1 6
Everything Bagel, 1 6
Muesli & Fruit Bagel, 1 5
Multigrain, 1 6
Onion Bagel, 1 5
Plain Bagel, 1 6
Poppy Seed Bagel, 1 6
Sesame Seed Bagel, 1 6
Whole Wheat & Honey Bagel, 1 5

CreamCheese

Herb & Garlic Cream Cheese, 3 Tbsp 4
Plain Cream Cheese, 3 Tbsp 4
Plain Light Cream Cheese, 3 Tbsp 3
Strawberry Light Cream Cheese, 3 Tbsp 3

Tim'sOwn™ Sandwiches

(on white bun)

Albacore Tuna Salad Sandwich, 1 8
Black Forest Ham & Swiss Sandwich, 1 13
Chunky Chicken Salad Sandwich, 1 8
Fireside Roast Beef Sandwich, 1 8
Garden Vegetable Sandwich, 1 10
Harvest Turkey Breast Sandwich, 1 8

POINTS

Soups

Beef Noodle, 1 bowl 3
Clam Chowder, 1 bowl 6
Cream of Broccoli Soup, 1 bowl 5
Cream of Mushroom Soup, 1 bowl 5
Hearty Vegetable Soup, 1 bowl 3
Italian Florentine, 1 serving 4
Minestrone Soup, 1 bowl 2
Tim's Own™ Chicken Noodle, 1 bowl 2
Turkey & Wild Rice Soup, 1 bowl 2
Vegetable Beef Barley Soup, 1 bowl 2

Chili&Beans

Chili, 1 bowl 5
Baked Beans (Quebec only), 1 bowl 6

Pies

Apple Pie, 1 slice (¼ pie) 11
Cherry Pie, 1 slice (¼ pie) 12
Lemon Meringue Pie, 1 slice (¼ pie) 10

Cakes

Black Forest Cake, with whipped cream, 1 slice 12
Caramel Topping for Coffee Cake, 1 Tbsp 1
Double Chocolate Delight, 1 slice 10
Tim's Own Coffee Cake, 1 slice 10

Tarts

Fresh Strawberry Tart, 1 4
Raisin Butter Tart, 1 8

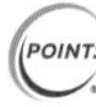

BakedGoods

Butter Croissant, 1 5
Cheese Croissant, 1 6
Cherry Cheese Danish, 1 9
Plain Tea Biscuit, 1 5
Raisin Tea Biscuit, 1 6
Southern Country Cranberry Biscuit, 1 10
Southern Country Raspberry Biscuit, 1 11

Cookies

Apple Cinnamon Cookie, 1 3
Chocolate Chunk Cookie, 1 4
Oatcake, 1 5
Oatmeal Raisin Cookie, 1 4
Peanut Butter Chocolate Chunk Cookie, 1 4
Peanut Butter Cookie, 1 4
Plain Macaroon, 1 4

Beverages

Café Mocha, 10 oz 3
English Toffee Cappuccino, 10 oz 3
French Vanilla Cappuccino, 10 oz 3
Hot Chocolate, 10 oz 4
Iced Cappuccino, made with 2% reduced-fat milk, 10 oz 3
Iced Cappuccino, made with cream, 10 oz 6

MealIdeas

1 bowl Tim's Own™ Chicken Noodle Soup
1 Butter Croissant

1 Honey Dip Yeast Donut
10 oz Café Mocha

1 Tim's Own™ Harvest Turkey Breast Sandwich (on white bun)
10 oz Iced Cappuccino (made with 2% reduced-fat milk)

Wendy's® (United States)

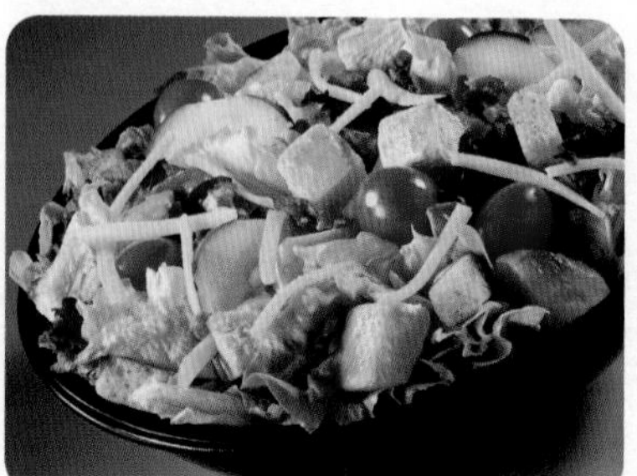

Burgers

Classic Single® Hamburger, plain, 1 8
Classic Single® Hamburger with Everything, 1 9
Big Bacon Classic®, 1 13
Jr. Hamburger, 1 6
Jr. Cheeseburger, 1 7
Jr. Cheeseburger Deluxe, 1 8
Jr. Bacon Cheeseburger, 1 9
Kids' Meal, Hamburger, 1 6
Kids' Meal, Cheeseburger, 1 7

Sandwiches

Chicken Breast Fillet Sandwich, 1 10
Chicken Club Sandwich, 1 11
Grilled Chicken Fillet Sandwich, 1 6
Spicy Chicken™ Sandwich, 1 9

French Fries

French Fries, 1 small serving 5
French Fries, 1 medium serving 8
Biggie® French Fries, 1 serving 10
Great Biggie® French Fries, 1 serving 12

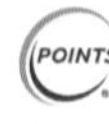

Baked Potatoes

Baked Potato, plain, 1 5
Bacon & Cheese Baked Potato, 1 13
Broccoli & Cheese Baked Potato, 1 10
Sour Cream & Chives Baked Potato, 1 7

Chili

Chili, 1 small serving (8 oz) 4
Chili, 1 large serving (12 oz) 6

Chicken Nuggets & Sauces

Chicken Nuggets, 5 pieces 6
Kids' Meal, Chicken Nuggets, 4 pieces 5
Barbecue Sauce, 1 packet (2 Tbsp) 1
Honey Mustard Sauce, 1 packet (2 Tbsp) 4
Sweet & Sour Sauce, 1 packet (2 Tbsp) 1

Garden Sensations™ Salads

Side Salad, 1 0
Caesar Side Salad, without dressing, 1 2
Chicken BLT Salad (Iceberg, Romaine, Spring Salad Mix, Cucumbers, Grape Tomatoes, Cheddar Cheese, Bacon Pieces, Diced Chicken), without Croutons and Honey Mustard Dressing, 1 7
Mandarin Chicken™ Salad (Iceberg, Romaine, Spring Salad Mix, Mandarin Oranges, Diced Chicken), without Roasted Almonds, Crispy Noodles and Oriental Sesame Dressing, 1 3

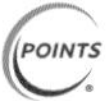

Spring Mix Salad (Iceberg, Romaine, Spring Salad Mix, Cucumbers, Grape Tomatoes, Red Onions, Carrots, Cheddar Cheese), without Pecans and House Vinaigrette Dressing, 1 4

Taco Salad, without Taco Chips, Sour Cream, and Salsa, 1 8

SaladDressings**&**Toppings

Blue Cheese Dressing, 1 packet (4 Tbsp) 8

Caesar Dressing, 1 packet (3 Tbsp) 4

Creamy Ranch, 1 packet 7

Fat Free French Style Dressing, 1 packet (4 Tbsp) 2

Honey Mustard Dressing, 1 packet 9

House Vinaigrette Dressing, 1 packet 6

Low Fat Honey Mustard, 1 packet 3

Oriental Sesame Dressing, 1 packet 7

Reduced Fat Creamy Ranch, 1 packet 3

Crispy Rice Noodles, 1 packet 1

Homestyle Garlic Croutons, 1 packet 2

Honey Roasted Pecans, 1 packet 3

Roasted Almonds, 1 packet 3

Salsa, 1 serving 1

Sour Cream, 1 packet 2

Taco Chips, 1 serving 5

Desserts

Frosty™ Dairy Dessert, 1 junior (6 oz) 4

Frosty™ Dairy Dessert, 1 small (12 oz) 7

Frosty™ Dairy Dessert, 1 medium (16 oz) 10

MealIdeas

1 Grilled Chicken Fillet Sandwich
1 Side Salad with
1 packet Fat Free French Style Dressing

1 Plain Baked Potato topped with
1 small serving Chili

1 Classic Single® Hamburger with Everything
1 Side Salad with
1 packet Fat Free French Style Dressing

Wendy's® (Canada)

POINTS

Hamburgers

Classic Single® Hamburger, plain, 1......8
Classic Single® Hamburger with Everything, 1......9
Big Bacon Classic®, 1......13
Jr. Hamburger Deluxe, 1......7
Jr. Cheeseburger Deluxe, 1......8
Jr. Bacon Cheeseburger, 1......9
Hamburger, Kids' Meal, 1......6
Cheeseburger, Kids' Meal, 1......7

Sandwiches

Chicken Breast Fillet, 1......9
Chicken Club Sandwich, 1......10
Grilled Chicken Sandwich, 1......6
Spicy Chicken Sandwich, 1......8

French Fries

French Fries, 1 small serving......7
Biggie® French Fries, 1 serving......10
Great Biggie™ French Fries, 1 serving......12

Baked Potatoes

Baked Potato, plain, 1......5
Bacon & Cheese Sauce Potato, 1......13
Broccoli & Cheese Sauce Potato, 1......10
Sour Cream & Chives Potato, 1......7

Chili

Chili, 1 small serving......4
Chili, 1 large serving......6

POINTS

Chicken Nuggets & Sauces

4 piece Kids' Meal, 4 pieces......4
Crispy Chicken Nuggets, 6 pieces......6
Barbecue Sauce, 1 packet (2 Tbsp)......1
Honey Mustard Sauce, 1 packet (2 Tbsp)......4

Garden Sensations™ Salads

Side Salad (Iceberg, Romaine, Cucumbers, Grape Tomatoes, Red Onions, Carrots), 1......0
Caesar Side Salad (Romaine, Parmesan Cheese, Bacon Pieces), 1......1
Chicken BLT Salad (Iceberg, Romaine, Spring Salad Mix, Cucumbers, Grape Tomatoes, Cheddar Cheese, Bacon Pieces, Diced Chicken), without Croutons and Honey Mustard Dressing, 1......7
Mandarin Chicken Salad (Iceberg, Romaine, Spring Salad Mix, Mandarin Oranges, Diced Chicken), without Roasted Almonds, Crispy Rice Noodles and Oriental Sesame Dressing, 1......3
Spring Mix Salad (Iceberg, Romaine, Spring Salad Mix, Cucumbers, Grape Tomatoes, Red Onions, Carrots, Cheddar Cheese), without Honey Roasted Pecans and House Vinaigrette Dressing, 1......4
Taco Supremo Salad (Iceberg, Romaine, Tomatoes, Red Onions, Cheddar Cheese, Wendy's Chili), 1......8

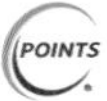

SaladDressings**&**Toppings

Caesar Dressing, 1 packet....4
Honey Mustard Dressing, 1 packet....9
House Vinaigrette Dressing, 1 packet....6
Oriental Sesame Dressing, 1 packet....7
Crispy Rice Noodles, 1 packet....1
Homestyle Garlic Croutons, 1 packet....1
Honey Roasted Pecans, 1 packet....3
Roasted Almonds, 1 packet....3
Salsa, 1....0
Sour Cream, 1....2
Taco Chips, 1 packet....5

Nachos

Chili & Cheese Nachos, 1....7

Frosty™Dairy**Dessert**

Frosty™ Dairy Dessert, 1 junior....4
Frosty™ Dairy Dessert, 1 small....7
Frosty™ Dairy Dessert, 1 medium....10

MealIdeas

1 plain Baked Potato, topped with
1 small serving Chili

6 pieces Crispy Chicken Nuggets with
1 packet Barbecue Sauce
1 junior Frosty™ Dairy Dessert

1 plain Classic Single® Hamburger
1 Side Salad with
1 packet Caesar Dressing

W.g. Grinders®

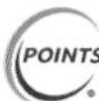

W.g.LighterSide

	POINTS
Bow Tie Pasta Salad, 1 serving	3
Chicken Noodle Soup, 1 cup	2
French Onion Soup, 1 cup	2
Minestrone Soup, 1 cup	1
Vegetable Soup, 1 cup	2
Light Chicken Salad Sandwich, 1	6
Light Turkey Sandwich, 1	7
Turkey Reuben Sandwich, 1	9

6-InchSandwiches

	POINTS
Baked Chicken Sandwich, 1	16
Chicken Parmesan Sandwich, 1	11
Ham and Cheese Sandwich, 1	15
Italian Sandwich, 1	11
Pizza Sandwich, 1	19
Tuna Sandwich, 1	10
Turkey Sandwich, 1	15

10-InchSandwiches

	POINTS
Baked Chicken Sandwich, 1	26
Chicken Parmesan Sandwich, 1	19
Ham and Cheese Sandwich, 1	25
Ham and Turkey Sandwich, 1	19
Spicy Sandwich, 1	23
Tuna Sandwich, 1	17
Turkey Reuben Sandwich, 1	16
Turkey Sandwich, 1	24
Veggie Sandwich, 1	12

Some Low-*POINT* Ideas

1 cup Minestrone Soup

each

1 cup Chicken Noodle Soup
1 cup French Onion Soup
1 cup Vegetable Soup

1 serving Bow Tie Pasta Salad

WHATABURGER®

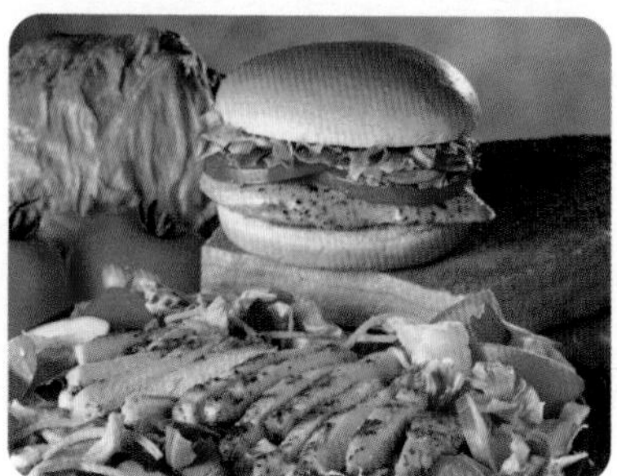

POINTS

Burgers&Sandwiches

JUSTABURGER®, with mustard, pickles, and onions, 1 7

WHATABURGER JR®, with mustard, pickles, onions, lettuce, and tomato, 1 7

WHATABURGER®, special request, on a small bun, without oil, with mustard, pickles, onions, lettuce, and tomato, 1 10

WHATABURGER®, with mustard, pickles, onions, lettuce, and tomato, 1 14

Double Meat, WHATABURGER®, with mustard, pickles, onions, lettuce, and tomato, 1 16

Grilled Chicken Sandwich, special request, on a small white bun, with lettuce & tomato, without oil, and mustard instead of salad dressing, 1 7

Grilled Chicken Sandwich, special request, with lettuce & tomato, without salad dressing, 1 9

POINTS

Grilled Chicken Sandwich, with salad dressing, lettuce, and tomato, 1 10

WHATACHICK'N® Sandwich on a wheat bun with salad dressing, lettuce & tomato, 1 11

WHATACHICK'N® Sandwich - Special Request on a small white bun, 1 11

ChickenStrips

Chicken Strips, 2 piece, 2 strips 9

Chicken Strips, 4 piece, 4 strips 19

Salads&SaladDressings

Chicken Strip Salad, 1 10

Chicken Strip Salad with Shredded Cheddar Cheese, 1 14

Chicken Strip Salad with Shredded Cheddar Cheese & Bacon, 1 16

Garden Salad, without dressing, 1 0

Garden Salad with shredded Cheddar Cheese, without dressing, 1 5

Garden Salad with shredded Cheddar Cheese & Bacon, 1 7

Grilled Chicken Salad, without dressing, 1 4

Grilled Chicken Salad with shredded Cheddar Cheese, without dressing, 1 9

Grilled Chicken Salad with shredded Cheddar Cheese & Bacon, 1 11

Low Fat Ranch Dressing, 2 oz 1

Low Fat Vinaigrette Dressing, 2 oz 1

Ranch Dressing, 2 oz 9

Thousand Island Dressing, 2 oz 4

POINTS

SideOrders

French Fries, 1 small serving 6
French Fries, 1 medium serving 9
French Fries, 1 large serving 11
Onion Rings, 1 medium serving 7
Onion Rings, 1 large serving 11
Peppered Gravy, 1 serving 1

Breakfast

Bacon & Egg Taquito, 1 9
Bacon & Egg Taquito with Cheese, 1 11
Biscuit with Egg & Cheese, 1 11
BREAKFAST-ON-A-BUN®, with Bacon, 1 9
BREAKFAST-ON-A-BUN®, with Sausage, 1 13
Egg Sandwich, 1 8
Hashbrown Sticks, 4 3
Pancakes with Bacon, without syrup or margarine, 1 serving (3 pancakes, 2 slices bacon) 14
Pancakes with Sausage, without syrup and margarine, 1 serving (3 pancakes, 1 sausage patty) 18
Pancakes, plain, 3 12
Potato & Egg Taquito, 1 9
Potato & Egg Taquito with Cheese, 1 10
Sausage & Egg Taquito, 1 10
Sausage & Egg Taquito with Cheese, 1 11

POINTS

Biscuits

Biscuit, plain, 1 7
Biscuit with Bacon, 1 9
Biscuit with Bacon, Egg, & Cheese, 1 13
Biscuit with Sausage Gravy, 1 12
Biscuit with Sausage, 1 13
Biscuit with Sausage, Egg, & Cheese, 1 17
Breakfast Platter (with 2 slices bacon, scrambled eggs, biscuit, and hashbrown sticks), 1 17
Breakfast Platter (with sausage patty, scrambled eggs, biscuit, and hashbrown sticks), 1 21

Desserts

Chocolate Chunk Cookie, 1 3
Cinnamon Roll, 1 10
White Chocolate Macadamia Nut Cookie, 1 6

Shakes

Chocolate Shake, 1 small 14
Chocolate Shake, 1 medium 21
Chocolate Shake, 1 large 29
Strawberry Shake, 1 small 14
Strawberry Shake, 1 medium 21
Strawberry Shake, 1 large 29
Vanilla Shake, 1 small 13
Vanilla Shake, 1 medium 19
Vanilla Shake, 1 large 26

MealIdeas

1 Grilled Chicken Salad with
2 oz Low Fat Ranch Dressing
1 Chocolate Chunk Cookie

1 JUSTABURGER®
1 Garden Salad with
2 oz Thousand Island Dressing

1 BREAKFAST-ON-A-BUN®, with Bacon
4 Hashbrown Sticks

White Castle®

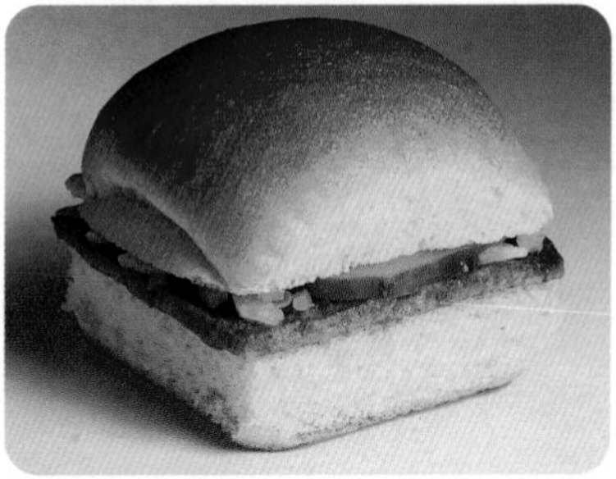

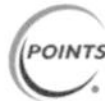

Burgers&Sandwiches

Hamburger, 1 3
Cheeseburger, 1 4
Double Hamburger, 1 5
Bacon Cheeseburger, 1 4
Double Cheeseburger, 1 7
Chicken Ring Sandwich, 1 5
Fish Sandwich, 1 4
Breakfast Sandwich (with egg, sausage, and cheese on a White Castle bun), 1 9

ChickenRings&SideOrders

Chicken Rings, 6 rings 5
French Fries, 1 small serving 2
Onion Rings, 8 rings 6
Cheese Sticks, 5 sticks 10

Shakes

Chocolate Shake, 1 6
Vanilla Shake, 1 6

MealIdeas

1 Bacon Cheeseburger
1 small serving French Fries

1 Hamburger
6 Chicken Rings

2 Cheeseburgers
1 small serving French Fries

Wienerschnitzel®

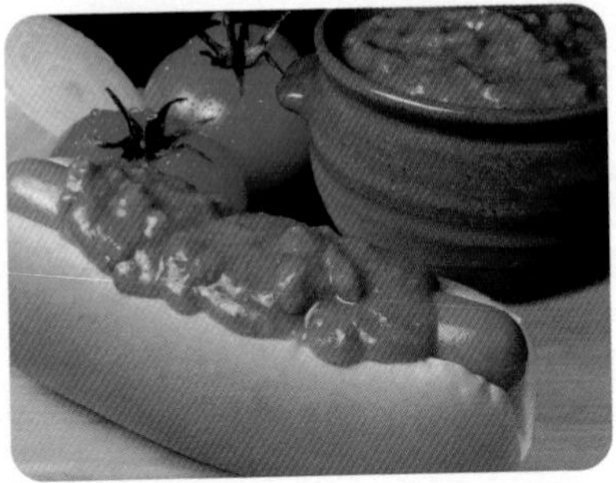

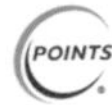

Burgers&Sandwich

Deluxe Burger, 1 15
Deluxe Cheeseburger, 1 16
Chili Cheeseburger, 1 16
Chicken Sandwich, 1 13

OriginalHotDogs&CornDog

Original Chili Dog, 1 7
Original Chili Cheese Dog, 1 9
Original Deluxe Dog, 1 7
Original Kraut Dog, 1 6
Original Mustard Dog, 1 6
Original Western Dog, 1 9
Corn Dog, 1 8

Fries

Fries, 1 regular serving 7
Fries, 1 large serving 10
Chili Cheese Fries, 1 serving 12

Breakfast

Breakfast Burrito, 1 15

Some Low-*POINT* Ideas

each

1 Original Mustard Dog
1 Original Kraut Dog

each

1 Original Chili Dog
1 Original Deluxe Dog
1 regular serving Fries

1 Corn Dog

Winchell's® Donuts

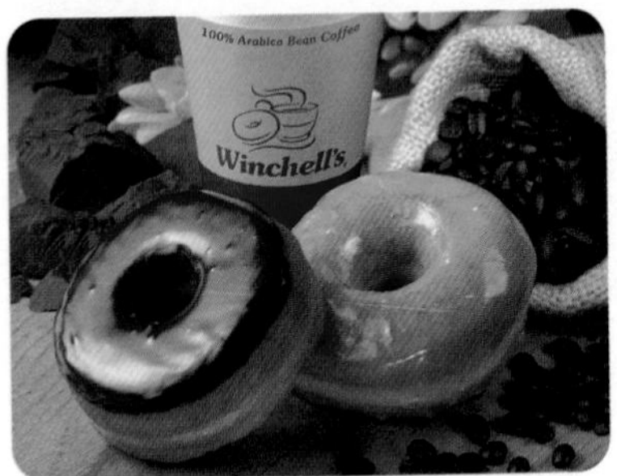

RaisedDonuts

Chocolate Bavarian, 1 8
Chocolate Rounds, 1 6
Chocolate Twist, 1 6
Glazed Jelly, 1 8
Glazed Rounds, 1 6
Glazed Twist, 1 6
Iced Bar, 1 6
Sugar Jelly, 1 8
Sugar Rounds, 1 6
Sugar Twist, 1 6

CakeDonuts

Cinnamon Crumb Cake, 1 7
Glazed Old Fashion, 1 7
Iced Cake, 1 6
Iced Donut Holes, 4 6
Iced Old Fashioned, 1 7
Plain Cake, 1 6

POINTS

OtherDonuts

Buttermilk Bar Glazed, 1 7
Iced French, 1 5

BakedProducts

Bagel, 1 6
Blueberry Muffin, 1 11
Bran Muffin, 1 10
Croissant, 1 7

Some Low-*POINT* Ideas

1 Iced French Donut

each

1 Chocolate Round or Twist Raised Donut
1 Glazed Round or Twist Raised Donut
1 Iced Bar Raised Donut
1 Sugar Round or Twist Raised Donut
1 Iced or Plain Cake Donut
4 Iced Donut Holes
1 Bagel

each

1 Cinnamon Crumb Cake Donut
1 Glazed or Iced Old Fashion Cake Donut
1 Buttermilk Bar Glazed Donut
1 Croissant

A
B
C

Local Favorites

POINTS

Abalone, fried, 3 oz ... 4

Ambrosia, ½ cup ... 2

Apple
- baked, 1 large ... 7
- candied, 1 large ... 10
- caramel, 1 large ... 9

Apple brown Betty, 1 cup ... 5

Apple crisp, ¾ cup ... 8

Bacon, lettuce, and tomato sandwich, 1 (9 oz) ... 12

Baked Alaska, 1 piece (2" wedge or 1⁄12 of 9" cake) ... 5

Banana bread, with or without nuts, 1 slice (5" x ¾") ... 5

Banana split, 1 (3 scoops ice cream, 1 banana, 3 Tbsp syrup, and ½ cup whipped cream) ... 19

Bananas Foster, 1 serving (2 scoops ice cream with ½ banana and ⅓ cup sauce) ... 16

Beans, baked, ½ cup ... 5

Beef, roast, open-faced sandwich with gravy, 1 (6 oz) ... 9

Beef goulash, 1 cup ... 8

Beef stew, 1 cup ... 5

Beef Stroganoff with noodles, 1 serving (1 cup stroganoff with 1 cup noodles) ... 15

Biscuit
- cheese, 1 (2" diameter) ... 5
- plain, 1 small (2" diameter) ... 3

Black Russian, 1 (3 fl oz) ... 5

Bloody Mary, 1 (5 fl oz) ... 2

Boston brown bread, 1 slice (3¾" x ½") ... 2

POINTS

Broccoli-rice casserole, 1 cup ... 5

Brownie, 1 (2" square) ... 5

Brunswick stew, 1½ cups ... 5

Buffalo wings, cooked, 3 (4½ oz) ... 9

Burgoo, 1 cup ... 4

Cake, with icing, 1 piece (1⁄12 of 9" layer cake or 3" square) ... 12

Carrot and raisin salad, ½ cup ... 7

Carrot cake, with cream cheese icing, 1 serving (1⁄12 of 9" layer cake or 3" square) ... 16

Cheese puffs, hot, 2 (½ oz each) ... 2

Cheese sandwich
- grilled, 1 (4 oz) ... 13
- with bacon, grilled, 1 (4¾ oz) ... 16

Cheese straws, 2 (2" long each) ... 2

Cheeseburger on bun, plain (without mayonnaise, lettuce, and tomato), 1 (6⅔ oz) ... 11

Cheesecake
- without fruit topping, 1 serving (1⁄16 of 10" cake) ... 10
- with fruit topping, 1 serving (1⁄16 of 10" cake) ... 10

Chef's salad
- without dressing, 4 cups ... 6
- with dressing, 4 cups ... 8

Chicken a la king, 1 cup ... 12

Chicken breast
- barbecued, with skin and bone, 1 (4½ oz) ... 6
- fried, with skin and bone, 1 (4½ oz) ... 11

Chicken drumstick
- barbecued, with skin and bone, 1 (1½ oz) ... 2
- fried, with skin and bone, 1 (1½ oz) ... 5

POINTS

Chicken Kiev, 1 serving (4" x 8") 18

Chicken-macaroni salad, 1 cup 6

Chicken paprika, 1 serving (1 breast or thigh with ½ cup sauce) 7

Chicken pieces (nugget-style), fried, 6 pieces (2" x ¾" each) 8

Chicken salad
- ½ cup 6
- Oriental, 2 cups 7

Chicken salad sandwich
- on reduced-calorie bread, 1 (5¼ oz) 8
- regular bread, 1 (5⅓ oz) 9

Chicken thigh
- barbecued, with skin and bone, 1 (3 oz) 5
- fried, with skin and bone, 1 (3 oz) 7

Chicken with dumplings
- without skin, 1 serving (3 oz chicken with 2 dumplings) 7
- with skin, 1 serving (3 oz chicken with 2 dumplings) 8

Chiffon pie, 1 slice (⅛ of 9" one-crust pie) 9

Chili dog on roll, 1 10

Cinnamon bun, 1 large (4 oz) 6

Club sandwich, 1 (8¾ oz) 15

Cobb salad (without dressing), 3 cups 10

Cobbler, fruit, any type, 1 cup 10

Coconut custard pie, 1 slice (⅛ of 9" one-crust pie) 9

Coconut shrimp, 4 jumbo 16

Coleslaw, ½ cup 4

Cookies
- bar, 1 (2" square) 3
- fortune, 1 (½ oz) 2
- gingerbread, 1 (2" diameter) 2
- macaroons, 2 (1 oz) 2

POINTS

Corn, on the grill, with butter, 1 (4 oz) 4

Corn bread, 1 piece (2" square) 3

Corn bread dressing, 1 cup 8

Corn casserole, ½ cup 8

Crab cakes, 2 (3" round each) 4

Crab puffs, 6 (1½" rounds) 5

Cream pie
- without fruit, 1 serving (⅛ of 9" one-crust pie) 9
- with fruit, 1 serving (⅛ of 9" one-crust pie) 9

Creamed chipped beef, 1 cup 11

Creamed chipped chicken, 1 cup 11

Creamed chipped turkey, 1 cup 11

Crème brulée, ¾ cup 11

Cruller
- 1 (2 oz) 6
- French, glazed, 1 (3" diameter) 4
- glazed, 1 (4" diameter) 6
- glazed, 1 long (approximately 5¼" x 2½" x 1½" high) 9

Custard, 1 cup 8

Custard pie, 1 slice (⅛ of 9" one-crust pie) 8

Daiquiri, 1 (3 fl oz) 3

Date-nut bread, 1 slice (5" x ½") 5

Doro wat, 1 cup 7

Doughnut holes, yeast, glazed, 2 (1 oz) 3

Doughnut
- cake-type, plain, 1 (3½" diameter) 6
- cake-type, sugared or glazed, 1 (3½" diameter) 6
- cake-type, with icing, 1 (3½" diameter) 7

Local Favorites

POINTS

Doughnut (con't)
- with crème filling, 1 (3½" x 2½" oval) 8
- yeast-type, glazed, 1 (4" diameter) 6
- yeast-type, with jelly filling, 1 (3½" x 2½" oval) 7

Duck, with fruit sauce, 1 serving (¼ duck with skin and ½ cup sauce) 13

Egg
- fried, 1 large 2
- scrambled, 2 or ½ cup 5

Egg salad, ½ cup 8

Egg salad sandwich, 1 (6 oz) 11

Eggs Benedict, 1 serving (2 English muffin halves with 2 eggs and ¼ cup Hollandaise sauce) 16

Fish
- baked, stuffed, 1 serving (6⅔ oz) 8
- fried, 1 fillet (6 oz) 12

Focaccia bread, 1 piece (¼ of 10" diameter) 6

Frankfurter on roll, plain, 1 (4 oz) 8

French toast, 2 slices (4½ oz) 7

Fritters, corn, 3 (2½" x 2" each) 5

Fudge, plain or with nuts, 1 piece (1" x 2") 3

Funnel cake, ½ cake (8" diameter) 12

Gelatin, fruit-flavored, ½ cup 2

Gin
- and tonic, 1 (6 fl oz) 3
- gimlet, 1 (2½ fl oz) 2

Gingerbread, 1 piece (3" square) 9

Green bean casserole, 1 cup 5

Greens, seasoned with bacon or salt pork, 1 cup 4

POINTS

Grinder sandwich, 1 (6" long) 6

Ham, glazed with pineapple, 1 serving (4 oz ham with ½ pineapple slice) 6

Ham and cheese sandwich
- 1 (4 oz) 9
- grilled, 1 (5 oz) 15

Hamburger on bun, plain (without mayonnaise, lettuce, and tomato), 1 (4½ oz) 9

Hero sandwich, 1 (6") 6

Highball
- made with unsweetened mixer, 1 (6 fl oz) 3
- made with sweetened mixer, 1 (6 fl oz) 4

Hoagie sandwich, 1 (6") 6

Honey bun, glazed, 1 (4" x 3" oval) 6

Honey roll, 1 (2 oz) 5

Hot chocolate
- without whipped topping, 1 cup 6
- with whipped topping, 1 cup 7

Hot dog on roll, plain, 1 (4 oz) 8

Ice cream soda, 12 fl oz 9

Ice cream sundae
- 1 scoop (½ cup) ice cream with syrup, nuts, and whipped topping 8
- 2 scoops (1 cup) ice cream with syrup, nuts, and whipped topping 11

Italian ice, water-type, ½ cup 1

Jalapeño bread, 1 slice (1½ oz) 2

Kabobs
- beef, 2 skewers (4½ oz) 8
- chicken, 2 skewers (4½ oz) 5
- fish, 2 skewers (4½ oz) 5
- lamb, 2 skewers (4½ oz) 8

POINTS

Key lime pie, 1 slice (1/8 of 9" one-crust pie) 13

King ranch chicken casserole, 1 cup ... 8

Lamb stew, 1 cup 5

Latte, made with fat-free milk
1 small (8 fl oz) 2
1 tall (12 fl oz) 2
1 grande (16 fl oz) 3

Latte, made with low-fat milk
1 small (8 fl oz) 3
1 tall (12 fl oz) 4
1 grande (16 fl oz) 5

Latte, made with whole milk
1 small (8 fl oz) 3
1 tall (12 fl oz) 5
1 grande (16 fl oz) 6

Lemonade, 1 cup 2

Liver
with bacon, 1 serving (2 slices [4 oz] liver with 2 slices bacon) 10
with onions, 1 serving (2 slices [4 oz] liver with 1/2 cup onions) 7

Lobster, steamed, 1 serving (1 1/4-pound lobster, or 4 1/2 oz lobster meat) 3

Lobster Newburg, 1 cup 14

Lobster roll sandwich, 1 (4 1/2 oz) 5

Lobster salad, 1/2 cup 4

Lobster salad sandwich, 1 (4 1/2 oz) 7

Lobster thermidor, 1 cup 14

Macaroni and cheese, 1 cup 9

Macaroni salad, 1/2 cup 6

Manhattan, 1 (2 fl oz) 3

Margarita, 1 (4 fl oz) 5

Martini, 1 (2 1/2 fl oz) 3

POINTS

Marzipan, 2 (1 oz) 4

Meat loaf, 1 slice (5/8" thick) 6

Mimosa, 1 (6 fl oz) 2

Mincemeat pie
without meat, 1 slice (1/8 of 9" two-crust pie) 13
with meat, 1 slice (1/8 of 9" two-crust pie) 12

Monte Cristo sandwich, 1 (3 3/4 oz) 6

Mushrooms, stuffed, 4 (2 3/4 oz) 3

Okra, fried, 1 cup 8

Old fashioned, 1 (2 fl oz) 3

Omelet
cheese, 1 (2-egg) 8
ham and cheese, 1 (2-egg) 9
herb or plain, 1 (2-egg) 6
vegetable, 1 (2-egg) 7

Onion, blooming, 1/4 (16" diameter) 6

Onion rings, fried, 4 (4" diameter each) 6

Oyster pie, 1 slice (1/8 of 9" pie) 9

Oyster po' boy, 1 (6") 17

Oysters, fried, 10 (5 oz) 7

Oysters Rockefeller, 4 (2 oz) 3

Pancake, 1 (4" diameter) 3

Paprikash, 1 serving (1 1/2 cups chicken mixture with 1/2 cup sauce) 9

Pasta salad, 1/2 cup 3

Pasta with garlic and oil, 1 cup 7

Peanut brittle, 1 oz 3

Pear, poached, 1 serving (1 pear with 2 Tbsp whipped cream) 5

Pepper, stuffed with beef and rice, 1 (7 3/4 oz) 8

Local Favorites

POINTS

Pepper steak, 6 oz 14

Philly cheese steak sandwich, 1 (9 oz) 13

Pie
- fruit, one-crust, 1 slice (⅛ of 9" pie) 6
- fruit, two-crust, 1 slice (⅛ of 9" pie) 9

Pierogies
- cabbage, 2 (3½" each) 7
- cheese, 2 (3½" each) 7
- meat, 2 (3½" each) 8
- potato, 2 (3½" each) 7

Pigs in blankets, 2 (1 oz) 6

Piña colada, 1 (6 fl oz) 7

Pineapple upside down cake, 1 slice (⅛ of 10" skillet cake) 10

Poor boy (po' boy), sandwich, 1 (6") 6

Popcorn
- buttered, popped, 3 cups 5
- movie, without butter, 3 cups 3

Pork, barbecue, 1 cup 8

Pot pie, chicken, 1 serving (8½ oz) 10

Potato, baked
- stuffed with bacon and cheese, 1 (9½ oz) 11
- stuffed with vegetables and cheese, 1 (13½ oz) 9

Potato, sweet, candied, ½ cup 4

Potato pancake, 1 (3¼ oz) 2

Potato salad
- ½ cup 7
- German, ½ cup 2
- hot, with ham, 1 cup 6

Potatoes
- garlic mashed, ½ cup 4
- hash brown, 1 cup 7
- home fried, 1 cup 5
- mashed, ½ cup 2
- scalloped, ½ cup 4

POINTS

Potatoes O'Brien, 1 cup 3

Pound cake, 1 slice (5" x 3" x 1") 8

Pretzels, soft, Philadelphia, 1 (4½" x 4") 3

Pudding
- any flavor, ½ cup 3
- any flavor, 1 cup 7
- bread, 1 cup 13
- corn, 1 cup 7
- Indian, 1 cup 7
- plum, 1 serving (½ cup with 1 Tbsp sauce) 9
- rice, 1 cup 8
- tapioca, 1 cup 5

Pumpkin bread, 1 slice (¾" thick) 7

Reuben sandwich, 1 (8 oz) 17

Rocky mountain oysters, 2 slices (1 oz each) 10

Runza, 1 (5½ oz) 8

Salad, mixed green, 1 cup 0

Salad Niçoise
- without dressing, 4 cups 8
- with dressing, 4 cups 18

Scallops
- fried, 20 small (3½ oz) 5

Scrapple, 1 slice (4½" x ¾" x ⅜" thick) 3

Screwdriver, 1 (6 fl oz) 3

Shrimp
- barbecued, 1 serving (4 large shrimp with ¼ cup sauce) 11
- broiled, stuffed, 6 large (6 oz) 18
- fried, 10 (5 oz) 8
- fried, stuffed, 6 large 9

Shrimp po' boy, 1 (6") 18

Shrimp puffs, 6 (1½" rounds) 5

Shrimp salad, ½ cup 3

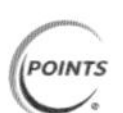

Shrimp salad sandwich, 1 (4½ oz)......7
Singapore sling, 1 serving (6 fl oz)......4
Sloppy Joe, 1 (6 oz)......7
Smoothie, 1 cup......2
Soufflé
cheese, 1 cup......5
fruit, ½ cup......4
Soup
broccoli-cheese, 1 cup......7
cabbage, 1 cup......1
cheddar cheese, 1 cup......9
chicken-noodle, 1 cup......3
cream of broccoli, 1 cup......6
cream of mushroom, 1 cup......9
cream of potato, 1 cup......2
cream of tomato, 1 cup......4
lobster bisque, 1 cup......4
Manhattan clam chowder, 1 cup......4
New England clam chowder, 1 cup......4
oxtail, 1 cup......1
Scotch broth, 1 cup......5
shark fin, 1 cup......2
tomato, 1 cup......2
vegetable, 1 cup......2
Spareribs, barbecued, 4 (4" long each)......8
Spinach salad, with dressing, 2 cups......7
Spinach soufflé, 1 cup......6
Spoon bread, ½ cup......4
Squid, fried, 3 oz......4
Steak
chicken fried (without gravy), 1 serving (6 oz)......13
chicken-fried (with cream gravy), 1 serving (6 oz with ¼ cup cream gravy)......17
Salisbury, 6 oz......11
Strawberry shortcake, 1 serving (1/12 of 9" cake or 1 filled individual shortcake)......7

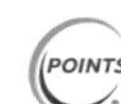

Stuffing, ½ cup......4
Submarine sandwich, 1 (6")......6
Succotash, cooked, 1 cup......4
Summer squash casserole, 1 cup......9
Swedish meatballs, 6 (1" diameter)......9
Sweet potato pie, 1 slice (⅛ of 9" pie)......9
Sweet roll, 1 large (4 oz)......5

Three-bean salad, ½ cup......4
Tomato, green, fried, 2 slices (1½" thick)......4
Tuna-macaroni salad, 1 cup......5
Tuna melt sandwich, 1 (5¾ oz)......9
Tuna-noodle casserole, 1 cup......9
Tuna salad, ½ cup......7
Tuna salad sandwich, 1 (6¼ oz)......10
Turkey-macaroni salad, 1 cup......5
Turnover, fruit, any type, 1 (3" x 1½")......5

Veal cutlet, breaded, fried, 4 oz......8
Vegetables
creamed (except cream-style corn), 1 cup......2
fried, 1 cup......4
sautéed, 1 cup......6
Vodka gimlet, 1 serving (2½ fl oz)......2

Waffle, any type, 1 (7" square)......5
Waldorf salad, ½ cup......4
Whiskey sour, 1 serving (3 fl oz)......2
Wine cooler, 8 fl oz......2
Wine spritzer, 8 fl oz......2

Zucchini bread, 1 slice (¾" thick)......5

Ethnic & Regional Favorites

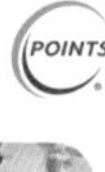

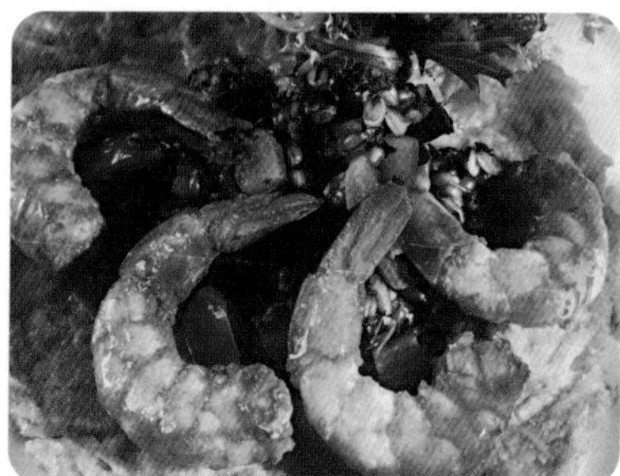

CajunFoods

POINTS

Bananas Foster, 1 serving (2 scoops ice cream with ½ banana and ⅓ cup sauce) 16

Barbecued shrimp, 1 serving (4 large shrimp with ¼ cup sauce) 11

Beans, red, and rice, 1 cup 5

Beignet, 1 (2") 2

Blackened
- chicken, 1 breast (3 oz) 7
- fish, 1 fillet (6 oz) 12
- steak, 6 oz 17

Crawfish pie, 1 slice (⅛ of 9" pie) 13

Creole
- chicken, without rice, 1 cup 6
- shrimp, without rice, 1 cup 4

Dirty rice, 1 cup 9

Etouffee
- crawfish, 1 cup 8
- shrimp, 1 cup 9

Green rice, 1 cup 6

Gumbo
- chicken, 1 cup 6
- seafood, 1 cup 5

Jambalaya
- chicken, with rice, 1½ cups 9
- fish, with rice, 1½ cups 9

Muffuletta, 1 (6") 20

Oyster pie, 1 slice (⅛ of 9" pie) 9

Poor boy (po' boy)
- sandwich, 1 (6") 6
- oyster, 1 (6") 17
- shrimp, 1 (6") 18

Praline, 1 (2½" diameter) 5

Remoulade
- sauce, 2 Tbsp 4
- shrimp, 1 serving (6 small shrimp with ¼ cup remoulade sauce) 9

Turtle soup, 1 cup 2

CanadianFoods

Donair
- 1 serving (4 oz meat with onion, tomato, and 2 Tbsp sauce) 14
- sauce, 2 Tbsp 2

Fish and brewis, 1 cup 13

Poutine, 1 serving (20 French fries with 2 oz cheese and ½ cup sauce) 17

Tortiere (Canadian meat pie), 1 slice (⅛ of 9" pie) 9

CaribbeanFoods

Chicken asopao, 1 serving (1 cup with 1 piece chicken) 8

Curry goat, 4 oz 5

Jamaican rice and peas, 1 cup 6

Jerk chicken breast, 1 large breast without skin 5

Plantain, fried, 1 cup 4

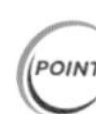
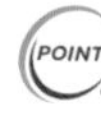
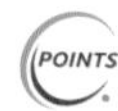

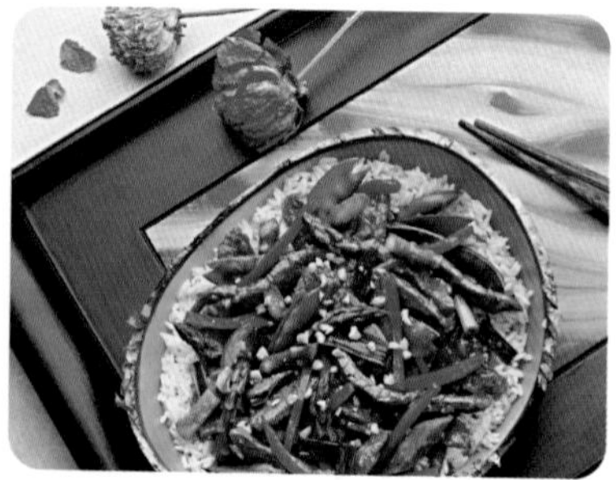

ChineseFoods

	POINTS
Beef and broccoli, 1 cup	4
Beef, orange-ginger, 1 cup	11
Black bean sauce, 1 tsp	0
Char shiu bao (roast pork bun), 1 (2 oz)	4
Chicken and broccoli, 1 cup	2
Chicken breast, five spice, with skin and bone, 1 (4½ oz)	7
Chicken leg, five spice, thigh and drumstick with skin and bone, 1 (6 oz)	9
Chicken with cashews, 1 cup	9
Chinese pancake, 1 (1 oz)	1
Chinese vegetables	
with beef, 1 cup	6
with chicken, 1 cup	5
with pork, 1 cup	7
with shrimp, 1 cup	4
with tofu, 1 cup	4
Chop suey	
beef, 1 cup	5
chicken, 1 cup	4
pork, 1 cup	4
vegetable, 1 cup	4
Chow mein	
beef, 1 cup	5
beef, chicken, or pork, canned, 1 cup	1
chicken, 1 cup	4
pork, 1 cup	5
Chow mein noodles, packaged, ½ cup	3
Crab Rangoon, 1 serving (1 large [4½"] or 5 mini)	5
Duck sauce, 1 Tbsp	1
Dumplings	
beef or pork, fried, 4 (6½ oz)	11
beef or pork, steamed, 4 (5¾ oz)	6
chicken, fried, 4 (6½ oz)	9
chicken, steamed, 4 (5¾ oz)	4
shrimp, fried, 4 (6½ oz)	9
shrimp, steamed, 4 (5¾ oz)	4
Egg foo yung	
beef, 1 (3" diameter)	4
chicken, 1 (3" diameter)	4
pork, 1 (3" diameter)	5
shrimp, 1 (3" diameter)	4
Egg roll wrapper, 1 (½ oz)	1
Egg roll	
beef, 1 (4½" long)	5
chicken, 1 (4½" long)	4
pork, 1 (4½" long)	5
shrimp, 1 (4½" long)	4
General Tso's chicken, 1 cup	15
Hunan beef, 1 cup	9
Kung Pao	
beef, 1 cup	10
chicken, 1 cup	8
pork, 1 cup	9
sauce, 2 Tbsp	1
shrimp, 1 cup	9

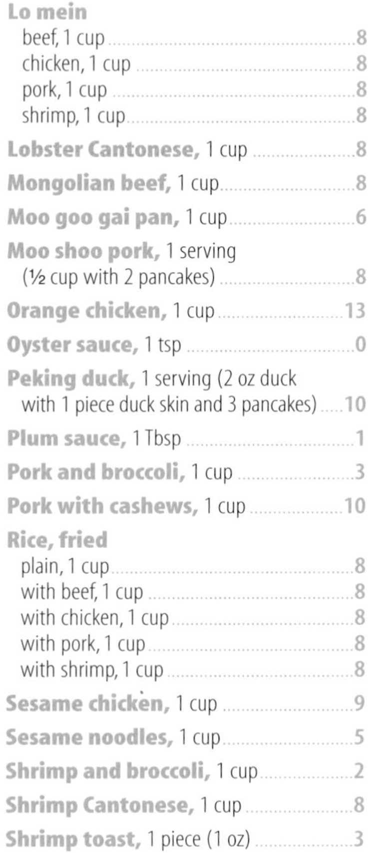

	POINTS
Lo mein	
beef, 1 cup	8
chicken, 1 cup	8
pork, 1 cup	8
shrimp, 1 cup	8
Lobster Cantonese, 1 cup	8
Mongolian beef, 1 cup	8
Moo goo gai pan, 1 cup	6
Moo shoo pork, 1 serving (½ cup with 2 pancakes)	8
Orange chicken, 1 cup	13
Oyster sauce, 1 tsp	0
Peking duck, 1 serving (2 oz duck with 1 piece duck skin and 3 pancakes)	10
Plum sauce, 1 Tbsp	1
Pork and broccoli, 1 cup	3
Pork with cashews, 1 cup	10
Rice, fried	
plain, 1 cup	8
with beef, 1 cup	8
with chicken, 1 cup	8
with pork, 1 cup	8
with shrimp, 1 cup	8
Sesame chicken, 1 cup	9
Sesame noodles, 1 cup	5
Shrimp and broccoli, 1 cup	2
Shrimp Cantonese, 1 cup	8
Shrimp toast, 1 piece (1 oz)	3

	POINTS
Soup	
egg drop, 1 cup	1
hot and sour, 1 cup	2
wonton, 1 serving (1 cup with 4 wontons)	4
Spareribs, Chinese, barbecued, 2 (4" long each)	4
Spring roll	
beef or pork, 1 (4½" long)	5
chicken, 1 (4½" long)	4
shrimp, 1 (4½" long)	4
Stir-fry	
beef with garlic or black bean sauce, 1 cup	8
broccoli, 1 cup	3
chicken with garlic or black bean sauce, 1 cup	7
pork with garlic or black bean sauce, 1 cup	8
shrimp with garlic or black bean sauce, 1 cup	7
Sweet and sour	
beef, 1 cup	12
chicken, 1 cup	10
pork, 1 cup	12
shrimp, 1 cup	10
sauce, 2 Tbsp	1
Wontons	
boiled, 6 (6 oz)	5
fried, 6 (4 oz)	11
Wonton skins (wrappers), 5 (3½" squares)	2

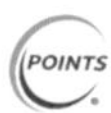

English/Irish**Foods**

Beef Wellington, 1 slice (3½" x 2½" x 1½") 12

Bubble and squeak, 1 cup 3

Carrots and parsnips, 1 cup 4

Colcannon, 1 cup 7

Crumpet, 1 (3" diameter) 3

Fadge, 1 piece (3¼ oz) 2

Fish and chips, 1 serving (5 oz fish fillet with 20 chips [French fries]) 15

Fruitcake, 1 slice (2½" x 1¾" x ½") 4

Irish brown stew, 1 cup 7

Irish coffee, 1 serving (6 fl oz with 2 tbsp whipped cream) 4

Irish soda bread, 1/12 of 8" round loaf 6

Popover, 2 (3" diameter) 4

Pudding
- bread, 1 cup 13
- plum, 1 serving (½ cup with 1 Tbsp sauce) 9
- Yorkshire, 1 piece (4" square) 6

Scone
- 1 small (1½ oz) 3
- 1 regular (2½ oz) 6

Shepherd's pie, 1 cup 9

Trifle, 1 cup 5

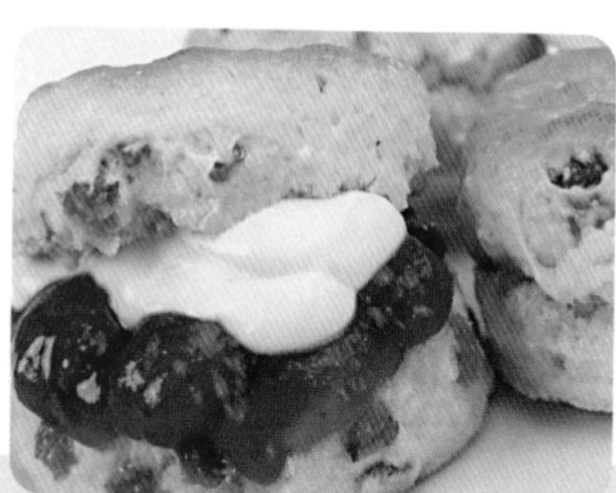

POINTS

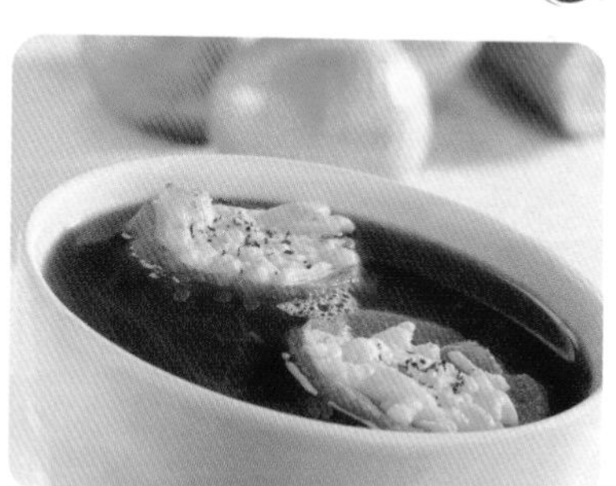

FrenchFoods

Baba au rhum, 1 (3¼ oz) 8

Bearnaise sauce, ¼ cup 8

Bechamel (white) sauce, ¼ cup 3

Beef Bourguignon, 1½ cups 20

Blanquette of veal, 2 cups 13

Bouillabaisse, 2 cups 7

Brioche, 1 slice (1 oz) 3

Cassoulet, 1 cup 11

Chicken cordon bleu, 1 piece (5½ oz) 13

Chocolate mousse, 1 cup 12

Coq au vin, 2 cups 13

Coquilles St. Jacques, 2 shells 8

Cream puff, 1 (2 oz) 7

Crème brulée, ¾ cup 11

Crème caramel, 1 cup 7

Crème fraiche, 2 Tbsp 3

Crêpes
- 1 (6" diameter) 2
- chicken, 2 (10½ oz) 12
- seafood, 2 (11 oz) 11
- Suzette, 2 (4¾ oz) 10

Ethnic & Regional Favorites

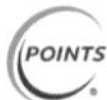

Croissant
- chocolate filled, 1 (5" long) ... 6
- plain, 1 (5" long) ... 5

Croque monsieur, 1 ... 11

Croquettes
- beef, 2 (2½ oz each) ... 10
- chicken, 2 (2½ oz each) ... 9

Duck a l'orange, 1serving (¼ duck with 2 Tbsp sauce) ... 13

Eclair, 1 (5¼ oz) ... 9

Escargots, 1serving (6 snails with 2 Tbsp butter) ... 7

Fish amandine, 1 fillet (6 oz) ... 13

Fish Veronique, 1 fillet (6 oz) ... 11

Fondue, cheese, 1serving (½ cup fondue with 2 oz bread) ... 12

Frog legs, fried, 2 (1 oz) ... 4

Hollandaise sauce, ¼ cup ... 8

Liver pâté, 1 slice (4¼" x 1½" x ½") ... 3

Mornay sauce, ¼ cup ... 3

Mussels Mariniere, 1serving (4 mussels with 3 Tbsp sauce) ... 5

Napoleon, 1piece (4½" x 2" x 1½") ... 14

Oysters Rockefeller, 4 (2 oz) ... 3

Peach melba, 1 serving (1 scoop [½ cup] ice cream with 2 peach halves and raspberry sauce) ... 7

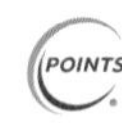

Petit fours, 2 (1¾" x 1½" x 1" each) ... 5

Petite marmite, 2 cups ... 7

Potatoes au gratin, 1 cup ... 13

Profiterole, 1 small (1 oz) ... 3

Quenelles, 8 (2½" x 1½" x ¾") ... 12

Quiche
- Lorraine, 1 serving (⅛ of 9" pie) ... 10
- vegetable, 1 serving (⅛ of 9" pie) ... 8

Ratatouille, 1 cup ... 4

Salad Niçoise
- without dressing, 4 cups ... 8
- with dressing, 4 cups ... 18

Sausage in brioche, 1 slice (2" thick) ... 15

Sorbet, any flavor, 1 scoop or ½ cup ... 2

Soufflé
- cheese, 1 cup ... 5
- fruit, ½ cup ... 4

Soup
- French onion au gratin, 1 cup ... 7
- vichyssoise, 1 cup ... 2

Steak au poivre, 1serving (6 oz steak with 1Tbsp sauce) ... 14

Tarte aux fruits
- 1 serving (⅛ of 9" tart) ... 8
- individual, 1 serving (4" tart) ... 11

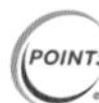

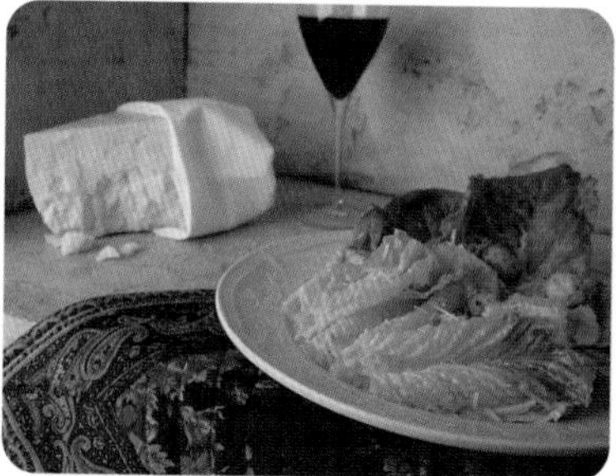

GreekFoods

Baklava, 1 piece (2" square) ... 4

Dolma, 4 (3½ oz) ... 4

Greek salad
- without dressing, 3 cups ... 2
- with dressing, 3 cups ... 9

Gyro, 1 (6") ... 15

Halvah, 1 piece (2" x 1¾" x 1") ... 5

Kataifi, 1 piece (2" long) ... 6

Moussaka, 1 piece (3" x 4") ... 12

Pastitsio, 1 piece (3¼" x 3") ... 13

Saganaki, 1 piece (1" x 2" x ½" thick) ... 6

Soup, avgolemono, 1 cup ... 4

Souvlaki
- 2 small skewers (4½ oz) ... 8
- 1 large skewer (4½ oz) ... 8
- sandwich, 1 (6½ oz) ... 8

Spanakopita
- 1 serving (3" square) ... 8
- 1 cup ... 8

Yogurt and cucumber salad, ½ cup ... 1

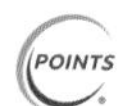

IndianFoods

Bean and lentil stew (Dal maharani), 1 cup ... 6

Chapati, 1 piece (5" diameter) ... 2

Chicken tikka, 4 oz ... 5

Curry
- beef, 1 cup ... 10
- Bengali fish, 1 serving (1 fillet [4½ oz] and 1 cup vegetables) ... 10
- chicken, 1 cup ... 10
- lamb, 1 cup ... 10

Dhansak, 1 cup ... 6

Indian coconut rice, 1 cup ... 5

Kashmiri (lamb meatballs), 6 (3½ oz) ... 11

Kheer, ½ cup ... 6

Korma
- chicken, 1 cup ... 14
- lamb, 1 cup ... 15
- vegetable, 1 cup ... 11

Lamb biryani, 1 cup ... 14

Mulligatawny soup, 1 cup ... 6

Naan, 1 piece (7" x 8" diameter) ... 4

Paratha, 1 serving (4" triangle) ... 3

Puris, 1 serving (4" diameter) ... 2

Raita, ½ cup ... 1

Samosa, 1 (2½" x 2½" x 3" triangle) ... 3

Tandoori
- chicken breast, without skin, 1 piece (4½ oz) ... 4
- chicken thigh, without skin, 1 piece (3 oz) ... 4

Vegetable fritters, 1 cup ... 10

Vegetable pakora, 1 (2" x 3") ... 3

Vindaloo
- chicken, 1 cup ... 8
- pork, 1 cup ... 9

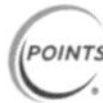

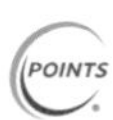

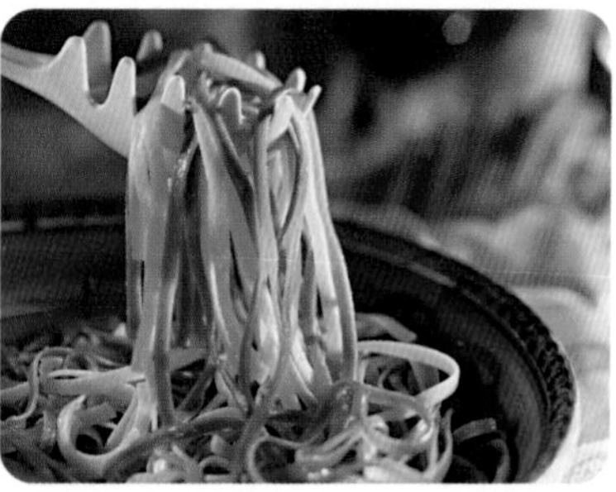

ItalianFoods

Amaretti cookie, 1 (1" diameter) 2

Artichokes, marinated ½ cup 3

Bolognese
- meat sauce, ½ cup 6
- spaghetti, 1 serving (1 cup spaghetti with ½ cup sauce) 10

Bruschetta, 1 slice (3 oz) 3

Caesar salad, 3 cups 7

Calamari, fried ½ cup 11

Calzone, 1 (5¼" x 6") 12

Cannelloni
- cheese, with meat sauce, 1 serving (2 shells with ½ cup sauce) 15
- cheese, with tomato sauce, 1 serving (2 shells with ½ cup sauce) 12
- meat, with cream sauce, 1 serving (2 shells with ½ cup sauce) 17
- meat, with tomato sauce, 1 serving (2 shells with ½ cup sauce) 14
- spinach and cheese, with cream sauce, 1 serving (2 shells with ½ cup sauce) ... 15
- spinach and cheese, with tomato sauce, 1 serving (2 shells with ½ cup sauce) ... 12

Cannoli, 1 (3½" long) 9

Caponata (eggplant appetizer), ¼ cup 1

Cappuccino, made with fat-free milk
- 1 small (8 fl oz) 1
- 1 tall (12 fl oz) 2
- 1 grande (16 fl oz) 2

Cappuccino, made with low-fat milk
- 1 small (8 fl oz) 2
- 1 tall (12 fl oz) 3
- 1 grande (16 fl oz) 3

Cappuccino, made with whole milk
- 1 small (8 fl oz) 2
- 1 tall (12 fl oz) 3
- 1 grande (16 fl oz) 4

Chicken cacciatore, 1 serving (1 half-breast or 1 thigh and leg) 10

Chicken marsala, without bone, 1 serving (4 oz) 15

Chicken parmigiana
- without sauce, 5½ oz 8
- with sauce, 1 serving (5 oz with ½ cup sauce) 10

Chicken tetrazzini, 1½ cups 14

Cioppino, 2 cups 13

Clams
- baked, 6 (2½ oz) 7
- fried, 1 cup 11

Clam sauce
- red, ½ cup 3
- white, ½ cup 5

Eggplant parmigiana
- without sauce, 1 serving (3" x 4") 11
- with sauce, 1 serving (3" x 4" with ½ cup Italian tomato sauce) 13

Fettuccine Alfredo, 1 cup 16

Garlic bread, 1 slice (1½ oz) 5

Gnocchi
- cheese, 1 cup 11
- potato, 1 cup 4
- spinach, 1 cup 12

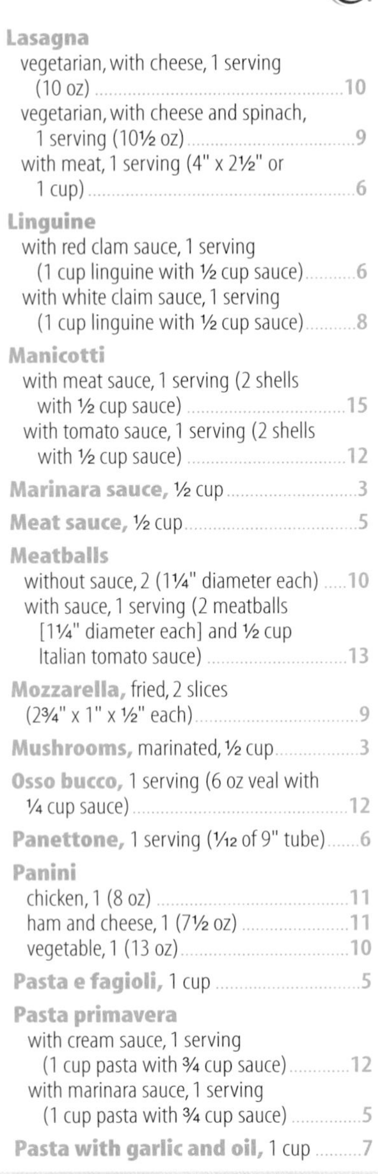

POINTS

Lasagna
- vegetarian, with cheese, 1 serving (10 oz) 10
- vegetarian, with cheese and spinach, 1 serving (10½ oz) 9
- with meat, 1 serving (4" x 2½" or 1 cup) 6

Linguine
- with red clam sauce, 1 serving (1 cup linguine with ½ cup sauce) 6
- with white claim sauce, 1 serving (1 cup linguine with ½ cup sauce) 8

Manicotti
- with meat sauce, 1 serving (2 shells with ½ cup sauce) 15
- with tomato sauce, 1 serving (2 shells with ½ cup sauce) 12

Marinara sauce, ½ cup 3

Meat sauce, ½ cup 5

Meatballs
- without sauce, 2 (1¼" diameter each) 10
- with sauce, 1 serving (2 meatballs [1¼" diameter each] and ½ cup Italian tomato sauce) 13

Mozzarella, fried, 2 slices (2¾" x 1" x ½" each) 9

Mushrooms, marinated, ½ cup 3

Osso bucco, 1 serving (6 oz veal with ¼ cup sauce) 12

Panettone, 1 serving (1⁄12 of 9" tube) 6

Panini
- chicken, 1 (8 oz) 11
- ham and cheese, 1 (7½ oz) 11
- vegetable, 1 (13 oz) 10

Pasta e fagioli, 1 cup 5

Pasta primavera
- with cream sauce, 1 serving (1 cup pasta with ¾ cup sauce) 12
- with marinara sauce, 1 serving (1 cup pasta with ¾ cup sauce) 5

Pasta with garlic and oil, 1 cup 7

POINTS

Penne a la vodka, 1 serving (1 cup pasta with ½ cup sauce) 7

Pesto sauce, 2 Tbsp 4

Pizza, restaurant-type, cheese
- thin crust, 1 small slice (⅛ of 12" or 1⁄12 of 16") 4
- thin crust, 1 large slice (⅛ of 16"-18") 6
- medium crust, 1 small slice (⅛ of 12" or 1⁄12 of 16") 4
- medium crust, 1 large slice (⅛ of 16"-18") 6
- deep-dish, 1 small slice (⅛ of 12" or 1⁄12 of 16") 5
- deep-dish, 1 large slice (⅛ of 16"-18") 8
- Sicilian, 1 slice (3" x 4") 7

Pizza, restaurant-type, one-meat topping
- thin crust, 1 small slice (⅛ of 12" or 1⁄12 of 16") 5
- thin crust, 1 large slice (⅛ of 16"-18") 7
- medium crust, 1 small slice (⅛ of 12" or 1⁄12 of 16") 6
- medium crust, 1 large slice (⅛ of 16"-18") 9
- deep-dish, 1 small slice (⅛ of 12" or 1⁄12 of 16") 7
- deep-dish, 1 large slice (⅛ of 16"-18") 11
- Sicilian, 1 slice (3" x 4") 9

Ravioli
- cheese, with tomato sauce, 1 serving (8 pieces or 1 cup with ½ cup sauce) 16
- cheese, without sauce, 1 serving (8 pieces or 1 cup) 13
- meat, with tomato sauce, 1 serving (8 pieces or 1 cup with ½ cup sauce) 14
- meat, without sauce, 1 serving (8 piece or 1 cup) 12

Risotto, ½ cup 5

Shrimp scampi, 9 medium 10

Soup
- lentil, 1 cup 3
- minestrone, 1 cup 4

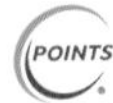

Spaghetti
carbonara, 1 cup 11
with marinara sauce, 1 serving (1 cup spaghetti with ½ cup sauce) 6
with meat sauce, 1 serving (1 cup spaghetti with ½ cup sauce) 9
with tomato sauce and meatballs, 1 serving (1 cup spaghetti, ½ cup sauce, and 2 meatballs) 16

Spumoni, ½ cup 7

Stromboli, 1 slice (1" thick) 4

Tirami-su, 1 piece (2¼" square) 10

Tomato and mozzarella salad, without dressing, 1 serving (2 large tomato slices with 2 oz cheese) 4

Tomato sauce, Italian, ½ cup 3

Tortellini
cheese, without sauce, 10 (⅔ cup) 3
meat, without sauce, 10 (⅔ cup) 3

Tortoni, 1 serving (2½ oz) 7

Turkey tetrazzini, 1½ cups 14

Veal marsala, 4 oz 13

Veal parmigiana
without sauce, 5½ oz 10
with sauce, 1 serving (5 oz with ½ cup tomato sauce) 12

Veal piccata, 2 slices (4 oz) 10

Veal scaloppine, 2 pieces (4½ oz) 8

Veal with peppers, 5 oz 11

Vitello tonnato, 1 serving (2 slices veal with ½ cup sauce) 16

Zabaglione, ½ cup 4

Zeppole, 1 (4" diameter) 6

Ziti, baked
without meat, 1 cup 6
with meat, 1 cup 9

Zuppa di pesce, 2 cups 11

Zuppa Inglese, 1 serving (1⁄16 of 10" cake) 8

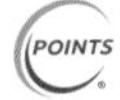

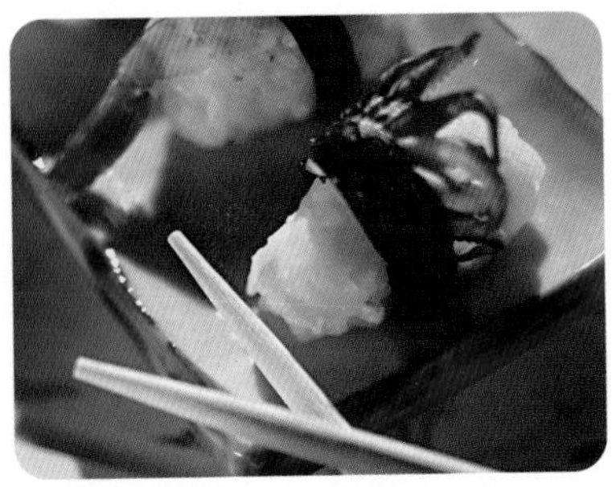

JapaneseFoods

Green tea ice cream, 1 scoop or ½ cup 3

Miso soup, 1 cup 2

Nebeyaki udon, 2 cups 5

Sashimi
any type except mackerel and salmon, 4 pieces (2 oz) 1
mackerel, 4 pieces (2 oz) 3
salmon, 4 pieces (2 oz) 2

Shabu shabu, 1 serving (4 oz beef, 2 oz tofu, and 1½ cups vegetables) 9

Suimono, 1 cup 1

Sukiyaki with sauce, 1 serving (2 cups with ¼ cup sauce) 12

Sunomono, ½ cup 0

Sushi
California roll, 4 pieces (1" high x 1¾" diameter) 3
maki (vegetables and rice rolled in seaweed), 4 pieces (5 oz) 2
nigiri (sliced raw fish over rice), 4 pieces (4 oz) 2
nori maki (raw fish and rice rolled in seaweed), 4 pieces (4½ oz) 2

Tempura
shrimp, 1 serving (4 jumbo shrimp) 12
vegetable, 1 cup 8

POINTS

Teppan yaki, 1½ cups 12

Teriyaki
beef, 2 slices (4 oz) 7
chicken, 2 slices (4 oz) 6
fish, 4 oz 5

Teriyaki sauce
1 Tbsp 0
¼ cup 1

Tonkatsu, ¾ cup 8

Yakitori, 1 skewer (7½ oz) 5

Yosenabe, 2 cups 4

JewishFoods

Bagel, any type, 1 small or ½ large (2 oz) 3

Bagel with cream cheese and lox, 1 large (6½ oz) 12

Bialy, 1 (3 oz) 5

Borscht, 1 serving (1 cup with 2 Tbsp sour cream) 4

Challah bread, 1 slice (5" x 3" x ¾") or 1½ oz 2

Cheese blintz, 1 (4¾ oz) 5

Chicken and meatball fricassee, 2 cups 9

Chicken in the pot, without skin, 2 cups 10

Cholent, 1 cup 4

Chopped liver, ¼ cup 5

Flanken, 2 slices (4 oz) 8

Fruit compote, ½ cup 3

Hamantaschen, 1 (3" diameter) 3

Haroset, ¼ cup 1

POINTS

Herring
chopped, ¼ cup 4
cooked, 1 oz 1
pickled, ½ cup 2

Honey cake, 1 slice (5" x 3" x 1") 7

Kasha varnishkes, 1 cup 5

Kishke, 1 small piece (¾ oz) 2

Kreplach
boiled, 2 pieces (4" x 3" x 3" each) 6
fried, 2 pieces (4" x 3" x 3" each) 7

Kugel
lukschen, without fruit, 1 piece (3" x 3¼") 5
lukschen, with fruit, 1 piece (3" x 3¼") 7
potato, 1 piece (3" x 3¼") 4

Mandelbrot, 1 slice (3" x 2" x ½") 5

Matzo, 1 board 2

Matzo brie, 1 serving (¼ of 10" round, or 1 cup) 5

Passover sponge cake, 1 serving (1⁄12 of 9" tube) 3

Pickled beets, ½ cup 1

Potato knish, 1 (3½" square) 6

Potato latkes, 2 (3½" diameter) 6

Rugalach, 1 piece (2½" x 1¼") 3

Schmaltz, 1 Tbsp 3

Soup
cabbage, 1 cup 1
chicken without matzo balls (broth only), 1 cup 0
chicken with matzo balls, 1 serving (1 cup soup with 2 [1½"] matzo balls) 3
mushroom-barley, 1 cup 3

Sponge cake, 1 serving (1⁄12 of 9" tube) 3

Stuffed cabbage, 2 (2" x 2½") 6

Vegetable tzimmes, ¾ cup 2

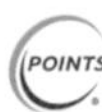

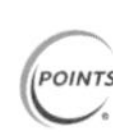

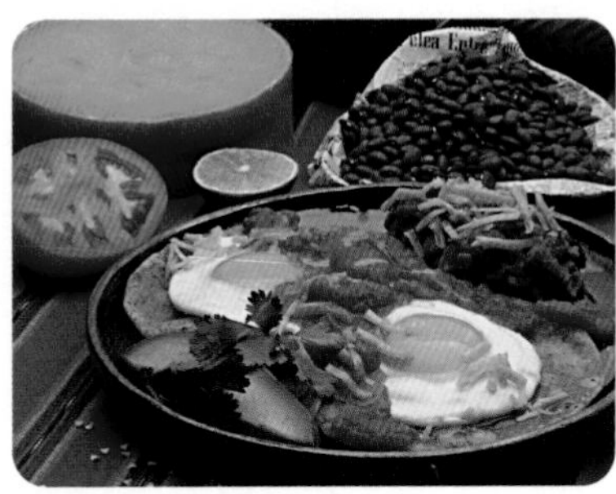

MexicanFoods

Arroz con pollo, 1 serving (3 oz chicken with 1½ cup rice) ... 13

Black bean and corn salsa, ½ cup ... 1

Burrito
- bean, 1 small (6") ... 5
- bean, 1 large (8") ... 8
- beef and cheese, 1 small (6") ... 5
- beef and cheese, 1 large (8") ... 8
- chicken and cheese, 1 small (6") ... 5
- chicken and cheese, 1 large (8") ... 7

Carne asada, 4 oz ... 10

Chalupa (pork and bean dish), 1 cup ... 6

Chicken adobo, 1 thigh (4 oz) ... 6

Chicken molé, 1 cup ... 8

Chili con queso, ¼ cup ... 5

Chili relleños, 2 (7½ oz) ... 18

Chili sauce
- green, ¼ cup ... 1
- red, ¼ cup ... 1

Chimichanga
- beef, 1 (3" x 3½") ... 11
- chicken, 1 (3" x 3½") ... 9

Chorizo, 1 link (5½" long) ... 12

Empanadas, 2 (3" diameter) ... 5

Enchiladas
- beef, 2 (10½ oz) ... 12
- cheese, 2 (8½ oz) ... 10
- chicken, 2 (10½ oz) ... 9
- pork, 2 (10½ oz) ... 12
- sour cream, 1 (5½ oz) ... 8

Fajitas
- beef, 2 (9 oz) ... 11
- chicken, 2 (8¾ oz) ... 8
- pork, 2 (10½ oz) ... 13
- shrimp, 2 (9 oz) ... 8

Flauta
- beef, 1 (6" x 1¼") ... 12
- chicken, 1 (6" x 1¼") ... 10
- pork, 1 (6" x 1¼") ... 11

Fried ice cream, 1 scoop or ½ cup ... 11

Gazpacho, 1 cup ... 3

Gordita, beef, 1 (3" diameter) ... 10

Guacamole, ¼ cup ... 2

Huevos rancheros, 1 serving (2 eggs on 2 tortillas) ... 14

Jalapeño poppers, 1 (1½ oz) ... 4

Menudo (beef tripe and hominy stew), 1 cup ... 6

Mexican 7-layer dip, ½ cup ... 3

Mexican coffee, 1 serving (6 fl oz with 2 Tbsp whipped cream) ... 4

Mexican corn bread, 1 piece (1⁄12 of 10" round) ... 7

Mexican wedding cookies, 2 (1½" wide each) ... 2

Molé poblano, ¼ cup ... 4

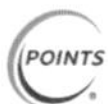

Nachos
beef, 4 (8½ oz) 13
cheese, 4 (3 oz) 8
cheese and bean, 4 (6½ oz) 9
chicken, 4 (8½ oz) 11
with cheese sauce, 1 serving (½ cup tortilla chips with ¼ cup cheese sauce) ... 5

Picadillo, 1 cup 10

Pico de gallo, ½ cup 1

Pozole, 1 cup 4

Quesadilla
beef, 1 serving (½ of 6" diameter) 7
cheese, 1 serving (½ of 6" diameter) 5
chicken, 1 serving (½ of 6" diameter) 6
vegetable, 1 serving (½ of 6" diameter) 6

Refried beans, ½ cup 3

Spanish rice, 1 cup 5

Sangria, 4 fl oz 2

Sofrito sauce, ½ cup 6

Sopaipillas, 2 (4" x 3" each) 3

Taco
beef, 1 (3½ oz) 5
breakfast, 1 (3¾ oz) 5
chicken, 1 (3½ oz) 4
fish, 1 (4¼ oz) 4
pork, 1 (3½ oz) 4

Tamale pie, 1 cup 11

Tamales, 2 (4" x 2") 9

Tortilla soup, 1 cup 6

Tostada
beef, 1 (8¼ oz) 10
chicken, 1 (8¼ oz) 8

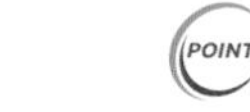

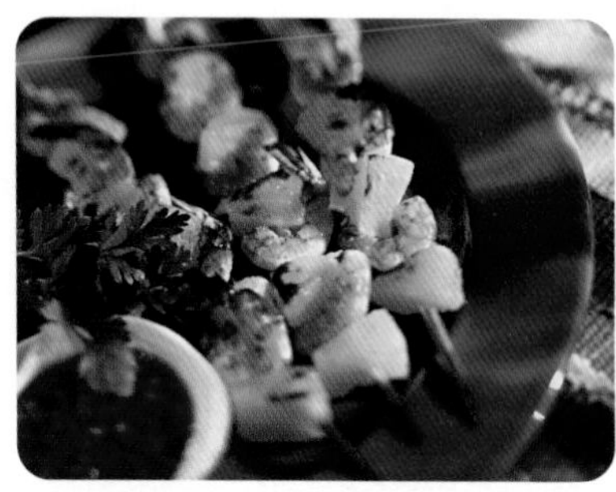

MiddleEastern**Foods**

Baba ganosh, ¼ cup 3

Falafel in pita, 1 large pita with 4 falafel patties 10

Falafel patties, 4 (2" diameter each) 7

Hummus, ¼ cup 3

Kibbe
baked, 3 pieces (1½" squares) 3
uncooked, ½ cup 4

Lavash, ¼ of 10" cracker 5

Rice pilaf, 1 cup 5

Sesame candy, 1 piece (2" x 1") 2

Shish kabob, 2 small skewers (4½ oz) 8

Tabouli, ½ cup 4

Tahini, 2 Tbsp 5

Yogurt and cucumber soup, 1 cup 2

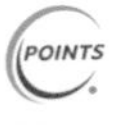

SpanishFoods

Black bean soup, 1 cup.....2

Ceviche, ½ cup.....2

Chili con carne
- without beans, 1 cup.....8
- with beans, 1 cup.....8

Flan, ¾ cup.....8

Paella, 1 cup.....7

Red snapper Veracruz, 1 serving (6 oz cooked fillet with ¾ cup sauce).....11

Spanish sauce, ½ cup.....2

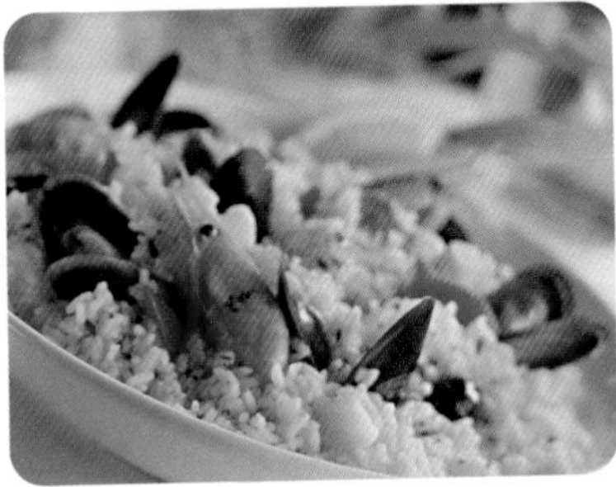

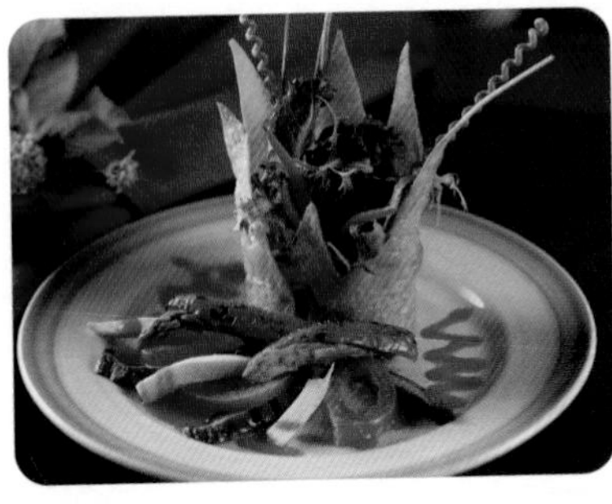

ThaiFoods

Green chicken curry (gaeng kheow wan gai), 1 cup.....7

Ginger chicken, 1 cup.....7

Mussaman beef curry, 1 cup.....19

Nam Prik, 1 Tbsp.....1

Pad Thai, 1 cup.....9

Peanut sauce, spicy, 2 Tbsp.....4

Satay
- beef, without peanut sauce, 2 skewers (3 oz).....5
- beef, with peanut sauce, 2 skewers with ¼ cup sauce.....11
- chicken, without peanut sauce, 2 skewers (3 oz).....3
- chicken, with peanut sauce, 2 skewers with ¼ cup sauce.....11

Seafood cakes (haw mok thalay), ¾ cup.....8

Soup
- hot and spicy chicken, 1 cup.....3
- Thai chicken coconut, 1 cup.....8

Thai beef salad, 1 cup.....14

Thai chicken with basil, without skin and bone, 1 breast (3¾ oz).....5

Thai coconut rice, 1 cup 8
Thai coffee or tea, 1 cup 7
Thai crisp noodles, 1 cup 8
Thai curry paste, 1 Tbsp 1
Thai paste, 2 Tbsp 2
Thai seafood salad, 2 cups 10
Tom yum kung, 1 cup 2

VietnameseFoods

Imperial roll, 1 (4½" long) 4
Lemon grass chicken, 1 cup 8
Nuoc cham, 1 Tbsp 0
Soup
  asparagus-crab, 1 cup 2
  Vietnamese beef-noodle, 1 cup 2
Vietnamese beef balls
  (thit bo vien), 6 (1½ oz) 2
Vietnamese spring roll, 1 (1¾ oz) 2
Vietnamese spring roll dipping
  sauce, 2 Tbsp 0

TrademarkAcknowledgments

A&W ALL AMERICAN FOOD: A&W is a registered trademark of A&W Restaurants, Inc. All American Food is a trademark of A&W Restaurants.

ARBY'S: ARBY'S®, ARBY-Q®, BIG MONTANA®, MARKET FRESH®, BRONCO BERRY SAUCE®, HORSEY SAUCE®, TANGY SOUTHWEST SAUCE®, and JALAPEÑO BITES® are registered trademarks of Arby's IP Holder Trust. ©2001, Arby's, Inc. Used with permission.

ATLANTA BREAD COMPANY: Atlanta Bread Company® is a registered trademark of Autumn Time, L.L.C., licensed to Atlanta Bread Company International.

AU BON PAIN: Au Bon Pain® and Mocha Blast® are registered trademarks of Au Bon Pain Co., Inc.

AUNT ANNE'S HAND-ROLLED SOFT PRETZELS: Auntie Anne's®, Glazin' Raisin®, and Dutch Ice® are registered trademarks of Auntie Anne's, Inc.

BACK YARD BURGERS: Great Little Burger® is a registered trademark of Back Yard Burgers.
Miz Grazi's™ is a trademark of Back Yard Burgers.
Gardenburger® is a registered trademark of Gardenburger Authentic Foods Company.

BAJA FRESH MEXICAN GRILL: Mini Quesa-dita™, Salsa Baja™ are trademarks of Fresh Enterprises, Inc.

BASKIN-ROBBINS: Baskin-Robbins®, Jamoca®, WORLD CLASS CHOCOLATE®, MAUI BROWNIE MADNESS®, and RASPBERRY CHEESE LOUISE® are registered trademarks of Baskin-Robbins, Inc. CAPPUCCINO BLAST™, CHOCOLATE BLAST™, and MOCHA CAPPUCCINO BLAST™ are trademarks of Baskin-Robbins, Inc.
OREO® is a registered trademark of KF Holdings, Inc. ©2003.

BIG BOY: Big Boy® is a registered trademark of Big Boy Restaurants International LLC.
©2002 Big Boy Restaurants, Inc. LLC.
Promise® is a registered trademark of Lipton.
Egg Beaters® is a registered trademark of Con Agra Brands, Inc.

BLIMPIE SUBS & SALADS: BLIMPIE® and BLIMPIE Best® are registered trademarks of Blimpie International, Inc.
MexiMax™, ChikMax™, and VegiMax™ are trademarks of Kellogg's/Morningstar Farms.

BOB EVANS: Bob Evans® is a registered trademark of Bob Evans Farms, Inc.
Egg Beaters® is a registered trademark of Con Agra Brands, Inc.

BOJANGLES': Bojangles'®, Bo Berry®, Bo Rounds®, Cajun Pintos®, and Dirty Rice® are registered trademarks of Bojangles' Restaurants, Inc. Cajun Spiced™ is a trademark of Bojangles' Restaurants, Inc.

BOSTON MARKET: Boston Market® is a registered trademark of Boston Market Corporation. Nestle® is a registered trademark of Nestle USA.
Oreo® is a registered trademark of Nabisco, Inc.

BREADSMITH: Breadsmith® is a registered trademark of Breadsmith Franchising, Inc.

BRUEGGER'S BAGELS: BRUEGGER'S BAGEL'S® , Bruegger's®, Herby Turkey®, and Leonardo Da Veggie® are registered trademarks of Bruegger's Corporation.

BURGER KING: BURGER KING®, WHOPPER JR.®, WHOPPER®, DOUBLE WHOPPER®, CHICKEN TENDERS®, and CROISSAN'WICH® are registered trademarks of Burger King Brands, Inc. BK FISK FILLET™ and BK VEGGIE™ are trademarks of Burger King Brands, Inc. BURGER KING® nutritional information used with permission from Burger King Brands, Inc.
KRAFT®, LIGHT DONE RIGHT®, and SIGNATURE are registered trademarks of the Kraft Foods North America, Inc.
COCA-COLA® and MINUTE MAID® are registered trademarks of The Coca-Cola Company.
The HERSHEY®'S is a registered trademark of Hershey Foods Corporation.

CARL'S JR.: Carl's Jr.®, Carl's Famous Star®, Super Star®, Western Bacon Cheeseburger®, CrissCut Fries®, Sunrise Sandwich®, and French Toast Dips® are registered trademarks of Carl Karcher Enterprises, Inc. Charbroiled BBQ Chicken Sandwich™, Charbroiled BBQ Club Sandwich™, Charbroiled Santa Fe Chicken Sandwich™, Carl's Catch Fish Sandwich™, Great Stuff™, Charbroiled Chicken Salad-To-Go™, and Garden Salad-To-Go™ are trademarks of Carl Karcher Enterprises, Inc.

CARVEL ICE CREAM BAKERY: Carvel®, Fizzlers®, Brown Bonnet®, and Flying Saucer® are registered trademarks of Carvel Corporation.

CHICK-FIL-A: Chick-fil-A®, Chick-n-Strips®, Cool Wrap® and Icedream® are registered trademarks of CFA Properties, Inc. Waffle Potato Fries™ is a trademark of CFA Properties, Inc.

CHURCHS CHICKEN: Churchs Chicken® and Jalapeño Cheese Bombers® are registered trademarks of Churchs Chicken. KRISPY TENDER STRIP™, Purple Pepper Sauce™, and Tender Crunchers™ are trademarks of Churchs Chicken.

COUSINS SUBS: Cousins Subs® is a registered trademark of Cousins Submarines, Inc.

DAIRY QUEEN: Dairy Queen®, DQ®, Brownie Earthquake®, Peanut Buster®, Buster Bar®, Chocolate Dilly®, Lemon DQ Freez'r®, Starkiss®, Misty®, Blizzard®, DQ Treatzza Pizza®, Brazier®, DQ Homestyle®, DQ Ultimate®, and Kid's Pick Nic! are registered trademarks of American Dairy Queen Corporation. Pecan Mudslide™, Chicken Strip Basket™ and Crispy Chicken™ are trademarks of American Dairy Queen Corporation.
Heath® is a registered trademark of Leaf, Inc.
M&M® is a registered trademark of Mars, Inc.
Oreo® is a registered trademark of Nabisco Ltd.
Skor® is a registered trademark used under license with permission of Hershey's Canada, Inc.
Smarties® is a registered trademark of Societe Des Nestle S.A.

D'ANGELO SANDWICH SHOPS: D'Angelo Sandwich Shops® and D'Angelo D'Lites® are registered trademarks of D'Angelo Sandwich Shops.

DEL TACO: Del Taco® and Macho Nachos® are registered trademarks of Del Taco, Inc. Del Cheeseburger™, Del Beef Burrito™, Del Classic Chicken Burrito™, Deluxe Combo Burrito™, Deluxe Del Beef Burrito™, Macho Beef Burrito™, Macho Chicken Burrito™, Macho Combo Burrito™, Big Fat Taco™, Big Fat Chicken Taco™, Big Fat Steak Taco™, Deluxe Taco Salad™, Deluxe Chili Cheese Fries™, and Macho Bacon & Egg Burrito™ are trademarks of Del Taco, Inc.

DENNY'S: Denny's®, Signature Skillets®, Chicken Fajita Skillet®, All-American Slam®, Corned Beef Hash Slam®, Farmer's Slam®, French Slam®, Lumberjack Slam®, Original Grand Slam Breakfast®, Scram Slam®, Slim Slam®, Ultimate Omelette®, Moons Over My Hammy®, The Super Bird®, Senior Belgian Waffle Slam®, Junior Grand Slam®, and Pizza Party are registered trademarks of Denny's Corp. Grand Slam Slugger™, FIT FARE™, Sampler™, Senior Omelette™, Senior Starter™, Burgerlicious™ Cheese Burgerlicious™, and Dennysaur™ are trademarks of Denny's Corp.
Egg Beaters® is a registered trademark of Con Agra Brands, Inc.
Oreo® is a registered trademark of Nabisco, Inc.
Quaker® is a registered trademark of The Quaker Oats Company.

DIPPIN' DOTS: Dippin' Dots® is a registered trademark of Dippin' Dots Inc.

DOMINO'S PIZZA: Domino's Pizza® is a registered trademark of Domino's Pizza PMC, Inc. All rights reserved. America's Favorite Pizza Feast™, Deluxe Pizza Feast™, ExtravaganZZa Pizza Feast™, Hawaiian Pizza Feast™, Meatzza Pizza Feast™, and Vegi Pizza Feast™ are trademarks of Domino's Pizza PMC, Inc. All rights reserved.

EAT'NPARK: Superburger® and Smiley® are registered trademarks of Eat'nPark Restaurants. Promise® is a registered trademark of Lipton.
Egg Beaters® is a registered trademark of Con Agra Brands, Inc.

EL POLLO LOCO: Pollo Bowl® is a registered trademark of El Pollo Loco 2003.

EL TORITO: EL TORITO® is a registered trademark of El Torito Restaurants, Inc. Cilantro-Pepita Dressing™ is a trademark of El Torito Restaurants, Inc.

FAZOLI'S: Fazoli's® is a registered trademark of Fazoli's Management, Inc.

FRESHËNS FROZEN TREATS: Freshëns® is a registered trademark of Yogurt Ventures U.S.A., Inc.

GODFATHER'S PIZZA: Godfather's Pizza® is a registered trademark of Godfather's Pizza, Inc.

HÄAGEN-DAZS SHOPS: Häagen-Dazs®, Cappuccino Commotion®, and Cookie Dough Dynamo® are registered trademarks of HDIP, Inc.
Bailey's® is a registered trademark of R & A Bailey & Co.

HARDEE'S: Hardee's®, Monster Burger®, and Super Star® are registered trademarks of Hardee's Food Systems, Inc. Famous Star™, Frisco™, Mushroom 'N' Swiss™, Big Roast Beef™, Fisherman's Fillet™, Hot Ham 'N' Cheese™, The Six Dollar Burger™, Crispy Curls™, Apple Cinnamon 'N' Raisin™, Biscuit 'N' Gravy™, Cinnamon 'N' Raisin™, Made From Scratch™, and Regular Hash Rounds™ are trademarks of Hardee's Food Systems, Inc.

JACK IN THE BOX: JACK IN THE BOX®, SOURDOUGH JACK®, JUMBO JACK®, JACK'S SPICY CHICKEN®, BREAKFAST JACK®, and EXTREME SAUSAGE® are registered trademarks of Jack in the Box, Inc.
Frank's Red Hot® is a registered trademark of Reckitt Benckiser.
Oreo® is a registered trademark of Nabisco, Inc.

JAMBA JUICE: Caribbean Passion®, Caribbean Craze®, Kiwi Berry Burner®, and PowerBoost® are registered trademarks of The Jamba Juice Company. Banana Berry™, Mango-A-Go-Go™, Orange Dream Machine™, Orange Mango Boom™, Orange-A-Peel™, Strawberries Wild™, and Juice Boost™ are trademarks of The Jamba Juice Company.

JERSEY MIKE'S SUBS: Jersey Mike's® Subs is a registered trademark of Jersey Mike's Franchise Systems, Inc.

JRECK SUBS: Jreck Subs® is a registered trademark of Jreck Subs, Inc.

KFC: KFC®, Original Recipe®, Tender Roast®, Triple Crunch®, and Colonel's Crispy Strips® are registered trademarks of KFC Corporation. KFC Extra Crispy™, Colonel's™ Pies, and Little Bucket™ Parfait are trademarks of KFC Corporation.
Hot Wings® is a registered trademark of Tyson Foods, Inc.

KRISPY KREME DOUGHNUTS: Krispy Kreme Doughnuts® is a registered trademark of HDN Development Corporation (a subsidiary of Krispy Kreme Doughnut Corporation).

KRYSTAL: Krystal® THE FAMOUS KRYSTAL®, CHEESE KRYSTAL®, DOUBLE KRYSTAL®, DOUBLE CHEESE KRYSTAL®, PLAIN PUP®, CORN PUP®, CHILI CHEESE PUP®, and KRYSTAL SUNRISER® are registered trademarks of the Krystal Company.

LITTLE CAESARS PIZZA: Little Caesars® Pizza, Meatsa®, Veggie!Veggie!®, Baby Pan!Pan!®, Italian Cheese Bread®, Crazy Bread®, and Crazy Sauce® are registered trademarks of Little Caesar Enterprises, Inc.

LONG JOHN SILVER'S: Long John Silver's®, Ultimate Fish Sandwich®, and Crumblies® are registered trademarks of Long John Silver's, Inc.

MAZZIO'S: MAZZIO'S®, Meatbuster®, and Supremebuster® are registered trademarks of Mazzio's Corporation.

McDONALD'S: McDonald's®, Quarter Pounder®, Big Mac®, Big 'N' Tasty®, Chicken McGrill®, Filet-O-Fish®, Super Size®, Chicken McNuggets®, Egg McMuffin®, and Sausage McMuffin®, and McDonaldland® are registered trademarks of McDonald's Corporation and its affiliates.
McFlurry™ is a trademark of McDonald's Corporation and its affiliates.
Butterfinger® and Nestle Crunch® are registered trademarks of Nestle U.S.A.
M&M® is a registered trademark of Mars, Inc.
Oreo® is a registered trademark of Nabisco, Inc.

MONICAL'S PIZZA: Monical's Pizza and Monical's® are registered trademarks of Monical's Pizza Corporation.

MR.GOODCENTS: Mr. Goodcents®, is a registered trademark of Mr. Goodcents Franchise System, Inc. Centsable Sub™, Mr. Goodcents Original™ , Penny Club™ and Centsational™ Size are trademarks of Mr. Goodcents Franchise System, Inc.

MRS. FIELDS: Mrs. Fields® is a registered trademark of Mrs. Fields Cookies, Inc. Nibbler™ is a trademark of Mrs. Fields Cookies, Inc.

PAPA JOHN'S: PAPA JOHN'S® is a registered trademark of Papa John's International, Inc. All the Meats™, Garden Special™, and The Works™ are trademarks of Papa John's International, Inc.

PAPA MURPHY'S TAKE 'N' BAKE PIZZA: Papa Murphy's® is a registered trademark of Papa Murphy's International, Inc. Chicago-Style Stuffed Pizza™, Chicken & Bacon Stuffed Pizza™, Hawaiian Pizza™, and Murphy's Combo™ are trademarks of Papa Murphy's International, Inc.

PICKERMAN'S SOUPS & SANDWICHES: The Pickerman's name is a registered trademark of Pickerman's Development Company, Inc.

PIZZA HUT: The Pizza Hut name, logos, and related marks are registered trademarks of Pizza Hut, Inc. and are used with permission.

PLANET SMOOTHIE: Planet Smoothie is a registered trademark of Planet Smoothie Franchises, Inc. Berry Bada-Bing™, Big Bang™, Billy Bob Banana™, Chocolate Chimp™, Chocolate Elvis™, Frozen Goat™, Grape Ape™, Hangover Over™, Leapin' Lizard™, Lunar Lemonade™, Mediterranean Monster™, Mr. Mongo-Chocolate™, Mr. Mongo-Strawberry™, PBJ™, Rasmanian Devil™, Road Runner™, Screamsicle™, Shag-a-delic™, Spazz™, The Last Mango™, Thelma & Louise™, Twig & Berries™, Two Piece Bikini-Chocolate™, Two Piece Bikini-Strawberry™, Vinnie Del Rocco™, Werewolf™, Yo' Adrienne™, and Zeus Juice™ are trademarks of Planet Smoothie Franchises, Inc.

PRETZEL TIME: Pretzel Time® is a registered trademark of Mrs. Fields Original Cookies, Inc.

ROUND TABLE PIZZA: Round Table®, Montague's All Meat Marvel®, Guinevere's Garden Delight®, and King Arthur's Supreme® are registered trademarks of Round Table Franchise Corporation. Chicken & Garlic Gourmet™, Chicken Rostadoro™, Gourmet Veggie™, Hearty Bacon Supreme™, Italian Garlic Supreme™, Maui Zaui™, Pepperoni Rostadoro™, Roastin' Toastin'™, Western BBQ Chicken™, Aloha Big Vinnie™, and Big Vinnie Pepperoni™ are trademarks of Round Table Franchise Corporation.

RYAN'S GRILL, BUFFET & BAKERY: Ryan's®, Mega Bar® and Fire Mountain® are registered trademarks of Ryan's Steakhouses, Inc.

SCHLOTZSKY'S DELI: Schlotszsky's® Deli, and Schlotzsky's® are registered trademarks of Schlotzsky's, Inc. Texas Schlotzsky's™ is a trademark of Schlotzsky's, Inc.

SIZZLER: Sizzler® is a registered trademark of Sizzler USA Franchise, Inc.

SMOOTHIE KING: Smoothie King®, Island Treat®, Lemon Twist Banana®, Lemon Twist Strawberry®, Light & Fluffy®, Muscle Punch®, Peanut Power®, Pep Upper®, Power Punch Plus®, Super Punch Plus®, and The Activator® are registered trademarks of Smoothie King Franchises, Inc. Angel Food™, Banana Boat™, Blackberry Dream™, Blueberry Heaven™, Caribbean Way™, Celestial Cherry High™, Cherry Picker™, Coconut Surprise™, Cranberry Cooler™, Cranberry Supreme™, Grape Expectations™, Grape Expectations II™, Hearty Apple™, Hulk™, Immune Builder™, Instant Vigor™, MangoFest™, Mo cuccino™, Muscle Punch Plus™, Orange Ka-Bam™, Peach Slice™, Peach Slice Plus™, Peanut Power Plus™, Pina Colada Island™, Pineapple Surf™, Power Punch™, Raspberry Sunrise™, Slim & Trim™, Strawberry Kiwi Breeze™, Strawberry X-Treme™, Super Punch™, Yogurt D-Lite™ Youth Fountain™, HeaterZ™, KingStix™, Berry Interesting™, Choc-A-Laka™, Gimme-Grape™, and Smarti-Tarti™ are trademarks of Smoothie King Franchises, Inc.

SONIC, AMERICA'S DRIVE-IN: Sonic®, Toaster®, Wacky Pack®, Ched 'R' Peppers®, Frozen Favorites®, Sonic Blast®, Fountain Favorites®, and Ocean Water® are registered trademarks of America's Drive-In Trust. SuperSonic™, Faves & Craves™, Sonic-Size™, CreamSlush™, and Premi-YUM™ are trademarks of America's Drive-In Trust.
Fritos® is a registered trademark of Frito-Lay, Inc.
M&M® is a registered trademark of Mars, Inc.
Oreo® is a registered trademark of Nabisco, Inc.
Reese's® is a registered trademark of the Hershey's Food Corporation.
Coca-Cola® is a registered trademark of The Coca-Cola Company.
Dr Pepper® is a registered trademark of Dr Pepper/Seven Up, Inc.

SOUPLANTATION: Souplantation® is a registered trademark of Garden Fresh Restaurant Corp.

STARBUCKS COFFEE: Starbucks Coffee®, Frappuccino®, and Tazoberry® are registered trademarks of Starbucks Coffee Company.

SUBWAY RESTAURANTS (UNITED STATES): SUBWAY®, Subway Club®, Veggie Delite®, Italian B.M.T.®, Subway Melt®, and Subway Seafood & Crab® are registered trademarks of Doctor's Associates, Inc. Cold Cut Trio™ is a trademark of Doctor's Associates, Inc.
M&M® is a registered trademark of Mars, Inc.

SUBWAY RESTAURANTS (CANADA): SUBWAY® and Italian B.M.T.® are registered trademarks of Doctor's Associates, Inc. Subway Club™, Veggie Delite™, Subway Melt™, and Subway Seafood and Crab™ are trademarks of Doctor's Associates, Inc.
M&M® is a registered trademark of Mars, Inc.

SWEET TOMATOES: Sweet Tomatoes® is a registered trademark of Garden Fresh Restaurant Corp.

TACO BELL: Taco Bell®, Taco Supreme®, DOUBLE DECKER®, Gordita Baja®, Gordita Supreme®, Burrito Supreme®, Enchirito®, MexiMelt®, and Nachos BellGrande® are registered trademarks of Taco Bell Corp. Zesty Chicken BORDER BOWL™ is a trademark of Taco Bell Corp.

TACO JOHN'S: Taco John's®, Taco Bravo®, Potato Olés®, Super Potatoes Olés®, and Mexi Rolls® are registered trademarks of Taco John's Seasonings Limited Partnership.

TACOTIME: TacoTime®, Big Juan®, Casita Burrito®, Mexi Fries®, and Cinnamon Crustos® are registered trademarks of TacoTime International, Inc.

TCBY: TCBY® is a registered trademark of TCBY Enterprises, Inc.

TIM HORTONS (UNITED STATES): Tim Hortons® and Timbits® is a registered trademark of T.H.D. Donut (Delaware), Inc. Tim's Own™ is a trademark of T.H.D. Donut (Delaware), Inc.

TIM HORTONS (CANADA): Tim Hortons® and Timbits® is a registered trademark of The TDL Group, Ltd. Tim's Own™ is a trademark of The TDL Group, Ltd.

WENDY'S: Wendy's®, Classic Single®, Big Bacon Classic®, Biggie®, and Great Biggie® are owned by Oldemark LLC and properly licensed to Wendy's International, Inc. Garden Sensations™, Mandarin Chicken™ and Frosty™ are owned by Oldemark LLC and properly licensed to Wendy's International, Inc.

W.G. GRINDERS: W.g.Grinders® is a registered trademark of Grinders, Inc.

WHATABURGER: WHATABURGER®, JUSTABURGER®, WHATABURGER JR.®, WHATACHICK'N®, and BREAKFAST-ON-A-BUN® are registered trademarks of WHATAPARTNERSHIP, L.P.

WHITE CASTLE: White Castle® is a registered trademark of White Castle Management, Inc.

WIENERSCHNITZEL: Wienerschnitzel® is a registered trademark of Galardi Group Franchise & Leasing, Inc.

WINCHELL'S DONUTS: Winchell's® is a registered trademark of Winchell's Donut Houses, Op. Co. L.P.

Photography Acknowledgments

Photographs courtesy of:

Arby's IP Holder Trust. ©2001, Arby's, Inc. Used with permission.

Autumn Time, L.L.C., licensed to Atlanta Bread Company International

Au Bon Pain Co., Inc.

Auntie Anne's, Inc.

Baskin-Robbins, Inc.

Big Boy Restaurants International LLC. ©2002 Big Boy Restaurants, Inc. LLC.

Blimpie International, Inc.

Bob Evans Farms, Inc.

Boston Market Corporation

Breadsmith Franchising, Inc.

Bruegger's Corporation

Burger King Brands, Inc.

Carl Karcher Enterprises, Inc.

Carvel Corporation

CFA Properties, Inc.

Churchs Chicken.

Cousins Submarines, Inc.

American Dairy Queen Corporation.

D'Angelo Sandwich Shops.

Domino's Pizza PMC, Inc. All rights reserved.

El Pollo Loco 2003.

El Torito Restaurants, Inc.

Fazoli's Management, Inc.

Yogurt Ventures U.S.A., Inc.

Godfather's Pizza, Inc.

HDIP, Inc.

Hardee's Food Systems, Inc.

Jack in the Box, Inc.

The Jamba Juice Company

Jersey Mike's Franchise Systems, Inc.

KFC Corporation

HDN Development Corporation (a subsidiary of Krispy Kreme Doughnut Corporation)

Little Caesar Enterprises, Inc.

Mr. Goodcents Franchise System, Inc.

Papa John's International, Inc.

Papa Murphy's International, Inc.

Mrs. Fields Original Cookies, Inc.

Schlotzsky's, Inc.

Smoothie King Franchises, Inc.

Garden Fresh Restaurant Corp.

Doctor's Associates, Inc.

Taco John's Seasonings Limited Partnership

TCBY Enterprises, Inc.

T.H.D. Donut (Delaware), Inc.

The TDL Group, Ltd.

Oldemark LLC, properly licensed to Wendy's International, Inc.

WHATAPARTNERSHIP, L.P.

White Castle Management, Inc.

Galardi Group Franchise & Leasing, Inc.

Winchell's Donut Houses, Op. Co. L.P.

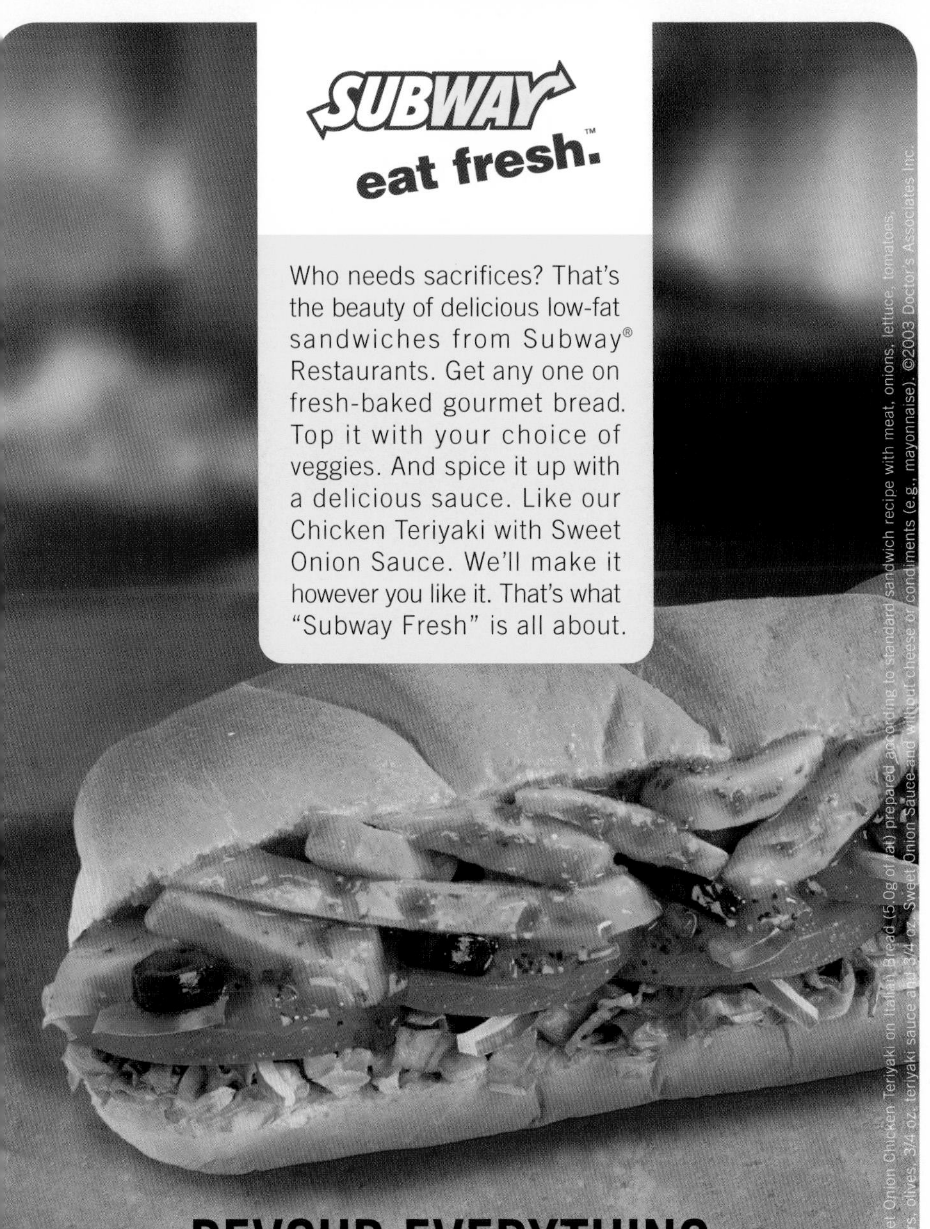
SUBWAY
eat fresh.™
Who needs sacrifices? That's the beauty of delicious low-fat sandwiches from Subway® Restaurants. Get any one on fresh-baked gourmet bread. Top it with your choice of veggies. And spice it up with a delicious sauce. Like our Chicken Teriyaki with Sweet Onion Sauce. We'll make it however you like it. That's what "Subway Fresh" is all about.
DEVOUR EVERYTHING.
SACRIFICE NOTHING.
Six-inch Sweet Onion Chicken Teriyaki on Italian Bread (5.0g of fat) prepared according to standard sandwich recipe with meat, onions, lettuce, tomatoes, green peppers, olives, 3/4 oz. teriyaki sauce and 3/4 oz. Sweet Onion Sauce and without cheese or condiments (e.g., mayonnaise). ©2003 Doctor's Associates Inc.

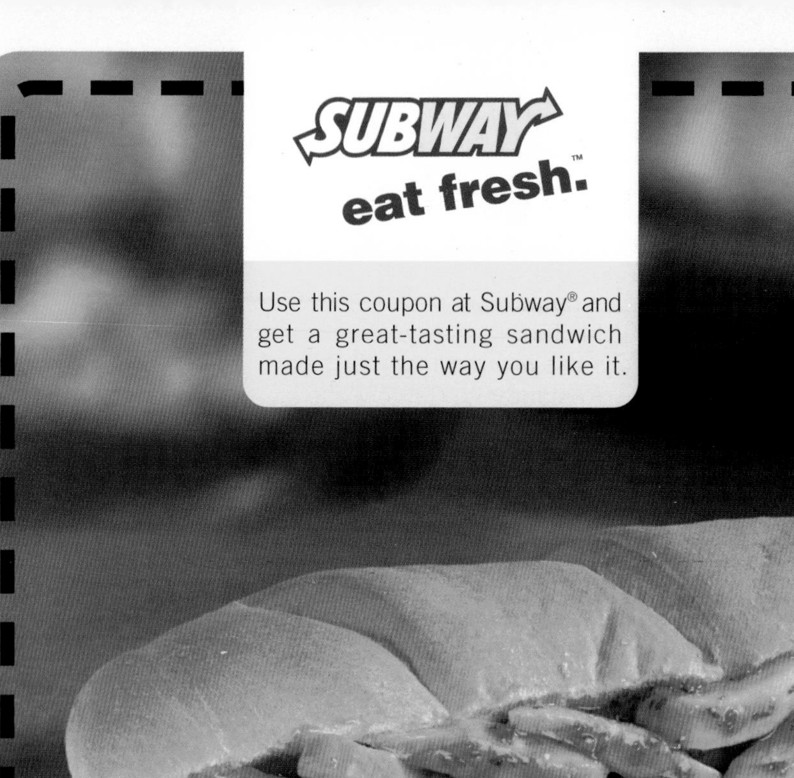
SUBWAY
eat fresh.™
Use this coupon at Subway® and get a great-tasting sandwich made just the way you like it.